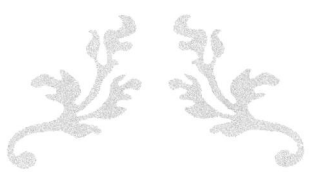

THIS WILL ONLY HURT A LITTLE...

A tourist guide to your Hospital Stay

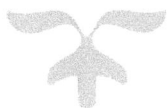

CONNIE CARSON-ROMANO RN

i

To my husband Michael who shares my adventures in life both

good and bad

And

To our wonderful daughter-in-law

Mandy

who is always there to make sure home is safe

while we are away

Table of Contents

One of the most frightening things we experience as human beings is when our bodies cease to function the way we expect them to, especially when the circumstances warrant hospitalization. Hospitals exist for us in a world of denial and wishful thinking that precludes the need of advanced medical care. Yet, the CDC reports that the average person in the United States has a one in 10 chance of requiring hospitalization in any given year. If you believe you are just going to the Emergency Department for outpatient treatment, think again. According to federal statistics your chances of ending up as a hospital admit from the emergency department are at 40%.

Human nature is to avoid things we do not understand. Hospitals lurk within this shadow realm of our thoughts until we need them. They are frightening places full of odd smells and populated with people who scurry around in funny clothes using a language that, while familiar in syntax, is foreign in content. Staff, in these places of frightening sensory stimulus, encourages the mystic perception that we feel towards these little understood houses of mystery.

Even Doctors, whom the general public perceive as being in control, are often confused and more than a little naïve about the happenings within the walls of our hospitals. Run by Administrators with little or no medical training and an eye towards profits and balanced budgets, they are staffed with caring professionals that are locked into a world that is anything but user friendly to either staff or patients. And that is before the well-meaning regulations set by a complex government system in an effort to control misuse of funds and provide universal healthcare. Add to this the Medicare limitations on reimbursement based on diagnosis which actually determine how long a patient should be allowed to stay in the hospital for a specific disease process and level of care required. This and the apparent ignorance of the human variables involved in medicine have contributed to the bed shortage in our nation. Hospitals want you to get well but on the predetermined schedule because they need your bed for the next patient in order to achieve their bottom dollar.

In a world of evolving medical care where the only aspect of care neglected seems to be the patients themselves, this book attempts to make the confusing world of hospitals a little more user friendly for the people whom they hope to serve. Having traveled extensively and lived in various areas of the country we recognize the regional differences in the focus on health care and thus the variations in the quality of care provided. Hopefully this book will answer some of your questions regarding hospitals no matter what area of the country you are from.

Used as an educational adjunct to the people who provide care for those patients, it can help make the caregiving a little easier for providers by explaining from a patients' point of view some of the frustrations of a hospital stay.

"It's always Worse at Midnight"

The worst has happened. The sickness hit you in the middle of the night and fearing the worst you dragged yourself out of bed and went to the local emergency room. After an hour wait in the lobby, where you became convinced that you should just go ahead and die right here in order to avoid more pain, a nurse came out and ushered you into the "triage room". She seemed cranky and you tried not to complain too much but somehow you seem to have made her mad anyway. She assured you, in no uncertain terms, that you were not the sickest person in this place and you should be glad you had to wait because it was a good thing you were not that sick. You avoided her eyes while you tried to rationalize that information in your mind. She handed you over to a technician of some sort who led you into an exam room, huffing and snorting because you were taking so long in your painful shuffling gait.

Following the technician into the exam room, a gown is thrown on the bed and you are told to undress, that someone will be in shortly. While the term 'shortly' does not describe the span of minutes that slowly ticks by, you are glad that you have been given a little time, while standing naked in the room, to figure out the snaps on the gown. Puzzles are your specialty. You figured out the Rubik's cube before anyone else, yet the gown snaps elude you and you finally lay down flat on the rock hard gurney draping the mystery gown over your exposed parts, feeling very chilled and finally understanding all the variations of vulnerability in the word naked.

The hospital definition of the short time frame finally passes as your buttocks grow numb and the Doctor walks into the room. You gratefully accept his adjustments to the back part of the bed although it causes the precariously placed gown to slither to the floor once again exposing parts best left covered. A few questions and the Doctor hands you back your failed gown. He tells you they are going to "run a few tests" as he snaps the computer shut and heads out the door.

Time slows and your feverish brain begins to contemplate the possibility of time travel as you spend hours being poked and prodded by complete strangers who touch your body in places your mother always told you to keep private. They draw blood; they zap you with radiation and sound waves, stick needles in your arm to which they add large bags of cold water, which give you worse chills and make you have to pee like the proverbial racehorse.

Your bladder feels like it is going to burst, yet when you call for help to let down the side of the bed, no one comes. When the nurse finally does comes in, instead of letting you up to go to the bathroom like a human being, she explains to you that in addition to all that cold fluid they put in your veins they gave you drugs that will make you fall down if you stand up. Your legs are thrown around like sacks of potatoes; they grab your privates and shove a tube up into your bladder, draining you into a bag that hangs embarrassingly at the side of the bed. The bag, which fills with what looks to be gallons of yellow pee is thrown

4

unceremoniously on top of you every time they drive you to another room for another test.

You are sick and exhausted and when the Doctor tells you they are going to keep you for a few days you think of all those movies with the quiet private beds, clean sheets, and pretty, sweet little nurses all dressed in white who come to comfort you as soon as you call. Compared to the horrors you have just been subjected to, this sounds like heaven and you agree wholeheartedly, signing reams of paper that may or may not give the hospital rights to your first-born. They tell you are now "an ED hold" and without explaining more, leave you alone for several hours more on the hard, torturous surface of the emergency room gurney during which you fantasize about the pleasure of the rest to come.

Drowsiness from that trouble causing pain medication takes hold and you start to drift into a fitful sleep. As you feel your head nod into semi-conscious relief, the door to your room bangs open causing you to wonder if they were watching and waiting for such a moment. A cheap floral fragrance enters the room causing your unsettled stomach to turn precariously. The odor is followed by and emanating from a perky young thing with frizzed hair and dangling earrings which bounce off her neck. She quizzes you on insurance and income, next of kin, and blatantly asks you if "should you die" you would like them to fix you or just let you go, as she smacks her gum loudly. The 'code status' question confuses you and you are a little slow at answering because you didn't think you were that sick. She rolls her eyes, popping her gum as she exits the room leaving the door standing wide open. You watch as the ED chaos runs past your door. What time is it?

Finally, when you think you can take no more, they once again throw the now full bag of urine, which is tugging at your inner privates, up on top of your lap for the world to enjoy as it merrily sloshes along with you. Weirdly you wonder what they would do if you put a goldfish in there. You are driven through what seems like miles of confusing corridors, up elevators, and past a room where someone is yelling for help. Anxiety builds as you are taken into a room with a person who never stops snoring even with the loud clashing and banging of your arriving gurney. Looking longingly at the awaiting bed and its cool crisp sheets you think you are tired enough to sleep through the snoring of your roommate. But before you can get up and crawl into the bed you have been thinking about for hours you are surrounded by hospital personnel, a giant piece of hard plastic is slid under you and you are yanked, sheets and all over onto the bed. Two CNAS roll you and flip you like a badly tossed pancake while you try to explain that you would rather do it yourself. One lays what appears to be a TV remote in the bed next to your bag of pee and then hangs the bag of pee down below where she drains it into a container. She writes Output 900 on the board and leaves the room before you can ask 900 what.

At this point, you find you are beginning not to care. You are so tired. You roll onto your side, fading into sleep. A low rumbling engine noise from beneath the bed rouses you as the bed starts inflating and rolling you from side to side. Thinking you have somehow broken the bed you push the button the aid told you to push "for assistance". No one comes. You lie on the rocking, rolling mattress and finally, in spite of the snoring King in the next bed and the seasickness your own bed is creating you drift off. Exhaustion, medication, and illness grab at your consciousness. Succumbing to the state of semi consciousness, you are suddenly roused from the beginnings of your fitful rest by a nurse dressed in a costume with yellow sponge personalities and odd shaped starfish on it, violently shaking your shoulder. "How come you pushed your call light? Do you need something?"

"Sleep...I need sleep...", you manage to mumble. "Well, then we don't want to push the red button, do we?" The vision in cartoon garb grumbles as she leaves your room. 'We? Where did "we" enter into this?', you wonder as you start to drift. The door is left open and, while you understand that hospitals are 24-hour facilities, you are amazed at the noises that form a cacophony with your snoring room partner. Bells, beeps, buzzer, staff with clunky shoes, happy staff that laughs all night, angry staff that complains all night, and the crazy person 3 doors down that alternately yells and moans 24 hours a day.

It is well after midnight and you finally manage little snippets of sleep. At the 4:00 am hour, some guy in the blue shirt swings into the room with a cleaning cart and gathers the garbage from the large metal garbage can, dragging it across the hard linoleum floor.

He closes the door behind him. Gratitude overwhelms you and you begin to drift again into the land of sleep, only to be awakened again at the 5:00 bloodletting. A phlebotomist who is young, perky and has had way too much coffee for this hour of the morning performs this early morning ritual. She is quick and efficient as she stabs needles into your arm digging for an elusive vein. Since they drained large quantities of blood last night in the ED you are a little surprised that this happens again but you are simply too tired to argue. In its sleep-deprived state, your mind assumes, in what seems like a reasonable fashion, that this in modern day makes up for the lack of an adequate supply of leeches. This perky vision wears a ceremonial white coat to signify her neutrality in the realm of ritualistic reduction of the arterial and venous volume, or so your mind now reasons. Adding, in what somehow seems rational, that this process is done at 5:00 am allowing for the tidal effects of the moon. You manage to mutter to Miss Perky that you would like her to close the door on the way out and she obliges as she bounces out of the room.

By now, it is close to 6:00 am and you find that this is the time designated for "the morning vitals". The antithesis of the perky phlebotomist slides into the room. This representative of modern medicine has obviously had NO coffee and is angry at the world. Grabbing your arm without preamble, she puts on an automatic blood pressure cuff, which has been set at max mode ten. Your fingers turn blue and your arm throbs as she holds your arm down and tells you that if you don't' hold still she will have to do it again. You comply and your fevered, exhausted brain tells you that the taking of the blood pressure, pulse, and temperature are mandatory at this hour because RA, the God of the sun chariot, is just beginning his travel across the sky, which, of course, makes for a more successful medical evaluation. You wonder if

8

perhaps she really works here as she speaks English in an accent that makes her unintelligible to the semi- conscious patient. Your snoring room fellow continues to taunt you with his unconscious state and you wonder how long he has been here.

Again, you begin to drowse off. And in pops "the nurse". She is not the nurse from the movies, the kind caring soul dressed all in white. This one is wearing Mickey Mouse clothing. Unfortunately for you, you wonder aloud if this is the pediatric ward. The Nurse pulls back and asks you if this confused state is normal for you. What does she mean by confused? You are not confused, just tired. You try to explain that you have been sick for days, and they tortured you last night and now all you want is to sleep. You tell her what you really want: The quiet room, like in the movies, and the happy little nurse, the one with white, squeaky shoes. She nods at you slowly in confirmation of her own understanding of some thought and slaps a yellow band on your wrist that defines you as a "fall risk". Pulling up the side rail on the bed, she programs something into the bed so that every time you turn over an alarm screeches in an ear-piercing trill. Nurse Mickey Mouse pats you on your hand and tells you in a voice you recognize as the one reserved for small children and crazy people that "It will be all right. " As she leaves the room, you try to call her back to explain that you are not crazy just sick and tired. Nurse Mickey puts her finger to her lips in a shushing posture and tells you to not get agitated or she will have to put the restraints on you. You lie back into the bed wondering what the restraints are and if you really are confused.

You have just about decided that you are feeling much better and don't really need a Doctor, just some sleep, preferably at home in your own bed, when the angry CNA slumps back into the room. Breakfast has arrived. Adjusting your bed into a position that thrusts your chest out as if at military attention, she pulls a table over you and slides a covered tray onto it. "Can you feed yourself?" She asks. Dumbfounded and afraid to say anything aloud you nod your head yes. As she grabs the cover from the food tray, a nauseating odor assails your nostrils. You feel your stomach lurch as you look at a mass of yellow next to a white biscuit with greyish white gravy on it. There is a bowl of white next to a glass of white, a small bowl of yellowish white, and some kind of off white spread. You recognize toast. There is toast. You reach for it over the yellow and white mass. There is also a child's box of orange juice and plastic mug of some brown liquid that smells like dishwater. The toast is dry and scratches your throat. You sit staring at the tray unable to escape its odors wishing for sleep until the CNA returns. "Not hungry?" She asks. You just stare at her. She repeats herself more slowly, "Are....you ....hungry?" You are not sure what "the restraints" mean but you are not willing to risk it and she is using that tone. You shake your head No and the ugly tray leaves just as the Dr. comes in. "I'll...be....back...to...give...you...a...nice...bed...bath." she says as she leaves the room. You stare after her in horror. No one has bathed you since you were two!

Your snoring roommate has somehow awakened in the midst of this chaos and has flicked his TV to the Today show. Matt Lauer's voice drowns out the Doctor as he comes into the room. He pauses and his lips move as he addresses the CNA but you cannot hear him because your roommate is laughing out loud at something Al Roker said to Savannah. "I see you've lost your appetite." says the Doctor holding your wrist and staring at the clock on the wall. This is just prior to informing you that the blood they drew this morning has somehow been mislabeled. Although they know it is your blood hospital policy won't allow them to re-label it so they will have to wait until tomorrow for another fasting blood level, which will determine if they need to do all the other tests he has ordered. Until then he says, he wants you to rest.

"Get well soon: The hospital needs your bed."

For 25 years I have worked in health care; initially as a Paramedic in a large city. Finding it more and more difficult to keep up with the younger medics and firefighters, I went to nursing school. After graduation, I specialized in Emergency and Critical Care working in various hospitals and settings. Eventually I accepted a position as a House Supervisor, a job that was well suited to the problem solving skills I developed as a Paramedic. It was at this hospital that I met the man who was to become my husband and who was then employed as one of the Emergency Room Physicians.

Married and happy we made commitments to grow old together. Growing older supposes specific patterns; and less than glowing health is one of those. My husband developed a serious illness several years ago. His condition, while allowing periods of health and freedom, requires ongoing medical treatment and, sometimes, hospitalizations. I, also, had a recurrence of a chronic debilitating illness. The education that I have received in the last few years as the wife of a patient and as a patient myself puts to shame my extensive training in nursing and the practices of my profession. Depersonalization of the individual has gone to new levels and the mechanics of patient care supersede the gentle, careful touch of a healer. Frustrated health care workers are locked in by a system that makes the caring peaceful environment needed for healing, a thing of the past.

Having worked in my profession for many years, I understand the psychological necessity of treating with denial some of the things we see and the emotional challenges of patients and their families that we deal with on a daily basis. To take home the emotions of every sad case we see could have serious emotional consequences for the providers in our field. Yet, somehow our profession needs to be called on the necessity of recognition of the person behind the disease process. He or she is not case # whatever...he (or she) is someone's family member.

Addressing the medical issues is a priority with any illness. However, the human element has been lost in the treatment of the body. As a Nursing Supervisor, I was called frequently to speak with angry patients and their families who felt frustrated at the lack of communication and demonstration of caring they encountered during their stay. More and more frequently, I found myself telling them that unfortunately Hospitals are for sick people, if you want to rest and get well, you have to go home.

All professionals like to think we have a good bedside manner but the truth is that our connection, more often than not, is disconnected from what the patient sees. The above story, while told in jest, has a frightening amount of truth to it. My own personal observations of my husband's treatment, my own treatment, and observations I have had as a supervisor all contribute to the retelling of a hospital admission from a patient's point of view. It is the perception of the patient and the

13

patients' family that can make all the difference in the world when it comes to a relaxed state that can allow for healing. Some of the solutions are simple, some more challenging but they all need to be addressed by the medical profession and the public.

More and more often the government is, by necessity, addressing some of the ongoing problems that exist in hospitals. Medicare is taking huge steps towards trying to force the system of hospitals to increase the quality of care provided to their patients and focus less on making a profit. New rules recently have begun to deny Medicare payment to hospitals that release patients so early that their recovery is jeopardized and they return within a month. This follows the rules that limit the number of hospital days they will reimburse based on diagnosis, which was forcing patients to be discharged before they were ready to go home. They are also denying payment to hospitals where patients who are being treated for one problem find themselves fighting off infections that are acquired in the hospital due to bad practices. Reimbursement is limited to the disease being treated and not the patient fighting that disease. It has become a frightening system.

I do understand that a large portion of the general public when admitted to a hospital, want to just turn over their care to the professionals. That is a wonderful fantasy but only a fantasy. There was a day and time when Dr. Marcus Welby, Dr. Kildare, and Dr. Quinn ruled in the fantasy world and the real world. The evolvement of medicine, with the creation of Hospitalists, eradication of CNA's and other support staff, and resulting duty load dumped on harried nurses and Doctors has created a world where trusting your care to a hospital without being involved yourself is dangerous.

I have attempted to lay out this book in inclusive chapters to make the reading and understanding more fluid. The chapters will follow what you can expect from admission following through to discharge. Not all of the problems mentioned exist in all areas but since it is difficult to know the quality of the hospital or the existing weakness of a facility until you are admitted as a patient, they have all been mentioned.

While national standards exist for hospitals they are all open to local interpretations resulting in an astonishing variance in the quality and type of care patients receive. Since my husband and I travel frequently, we have had the...ok we will call it opportunity, to see hospitals from New Jersey to California, literally coast to coast. It has been an eye opening experience.

My husband, a retired Emergency Room physician, and I, have between us, close to 6 decades of experience in dealing with patients, hospitals, and professional ancillary personnel. Even with that, we have often found ourselves at a loss when fighting our way through the systems. The frustration that we have felt with our medical system as trained, experienced professionals made the realization of how frightening it must be to enter the hospital system with no idea of what to expect from the providers or what they will expect from you, very real. Therefore, we are using our experience as providers and experiences as patients to create a basic (and hopefully entertaining) hand book on how to navigate your way through your hospital stay.

Patient Rights, Paperwork Wrongs and Hospital Beginnings

It is only fair to start this chapter out with the warning that it is next to impossible to write a chapter on hospital paperwork and history that is tantalizing and exciting. I will, therefore, merely attempt to make it readable. Please bear in mind the subject matter and then hang in there. Is it important to know what all that paperwork says? I think so or I would not have done the research and reading required for this chapter. I found it all extremely dull. If you find it too boring you could probably just skip this chapter or scan through it for the good parts but it does contain information that you may need to know during your stay. Most importantly your rights as a patient. So, since the material contained in that paperwork is important I will do my best to make this "only hurt a little."

The practice of medicine has always been a bit of a mystery to most people. The study of the human body and the processes that interfere with the proper functioning of it are challenging and involved. There have always been in our societies some person or group of persons who were designated as the medical caregiver. Oft times the role is combined with the spirituality of the community in deference to the mysterious functioning of the human body and the mystical denial of the possibility of death. No matter the practice that has existed there has always been somewhat of a division between those who try to understand and manipulate our physiology and the balance of society which feels safer in not knowing.

Human bodies are incredible things. The processes that happen inside of us every day are complicated, confusing, and mysterious even in this day of modern science. As fascinating as it is to watch the intricate processes that keep us alive it is also frightening to watch the process cease to function properly. After years of working in medicine, I think most people feel safer not knowing too much about the workings of the body. We need to trust our bodies to function smoothly. Therefore, we hand our medical care to the gifted few who strive to understand it and control it. That also creates a dilemma when our bodies do fail us and we have to seek out someone to help us fix it.

Hospitals have been around for centuries. The first documented hospitals were affiliated with religious sects in Egypt and Greece. It is not surprising that the mystery of the human body should be assigned to the mysteries of religion, and that the quality of the care received at these facilities fluctuates with the flow of religion being practiced. The symbiosis of the art of healing from the church and religious influences has been ongoing over the centuries. The perceived mystery of the transpiring events in the hospital will remain with us as long as people remained frightened of illness and injury. Denial that it can happen to you creates a fertile field for ignorance into the workings of the medical community. Simply put, people do not want to know about Doctors and medicine until they, or someone they love, is in need of the services of medical providers.

Some progress has been made into 'guarantees' that will make these places less frightening. Federal laws are in place that guarantee you specific medical rights. Yet progress is slow in the evolution of these laws and complicated by the ridiculous animosity that exists between branches of our governing powers.

The history of hospitals in the United States is as diverse as our culture. While most 'modern' hospitals initially were designed by various churches as a form of not for profit charity, there are also hospitals owned and operated by the government, by schools, and by private entities. The diversity of the fundamentals of development of these varied facilities attests strongly to the varied levels of care received at different ones. Privately run 'for profit' hospitals that refused emergency care to the poor, performed experimentation on prisoners and those unable to speak for themselves, lack of privacy, and a variety of other wrongs that grew over the years have created a need for regulation. It has been a slow process but progress is being made.

I wish I could tell you here that all of the concerns of a patient in a hospital have been addressed on the federal level. However, as medicine is an evolving practice the rights that need to be protected are changing as fast, if not faster, than the laws can be written.

In 1973, the American Hospital Association published the first of many Patients' Bill of rights. While it has changed over the years, the fundamentals are still there. You can access the complete document on line at www.aha.org/resource/ptbillofrights.html if you wish to read it in its entirety or retain a copy with which to scare your nurse by leaving it lie around in your room. It also can be successfully substituted for any sleep aid.

As I said earlier, the diversity of documents proclaiming themselves to be a patient's bill of rights can be intimidating. This diversity is encouraged by AHA to make it readable to all classes and schools of patients. Your best bet for understanding these in depth is to do an internet search for your local region or state. With all of the recent interest generated in the healthcare industry, more and more local governments are pursuing ways to help people better control their own environment while in the hospital. For instance, the California Hospital Association has a very understandable document online that combines a patient bill of rights with laws specifically written into the regulatory document for California medical care known as title 22.

The latest federal level Patients' bill of rights was created along with the Affordable Care Act and addresses not only hospital stays but also insurance issues that patients may have to address.

The first right on this list is one that is frequently violated due to the hurried nature the medical community has adopted in its rush to make the dollars fit the costs. It states that the patient has the right to obtain from physicians and other direct caregivers understandable information about their diagnosis, treatment, and prognosis. It takes time and patience to explain disease process to someone who has never had medical training. Diagnosis that is more complicated may not be completely understood by the physician or the nurse. In such a case, honesty is the best policy. Admitting to a patient who has entrusted you with their care that you do not understand their problem completely is a difficult thing to do but completely acceptable if an effort is then made to provide the patient with that information. Medicine is a complicated field that supports an army of specialties that study varied disease processes. No Doctor knows everything about every disease but they can look it up or refer you to someone who does know.

This right to know and understand is of course limited in emergency situations when explaining things in detail could endanger the life of the patient. However, even treatment in an emergency situation should be explained to you after the fact.

You also have the right to make a choice in your health care providers; which Doctor you see, which Hospital you go to, which insurance you use. This, of course, is where a patient's true power lies; in the capitalistic forum that supports our health care system. It is your responsibility to make sure that you choose wisely. Make sure that your Doctor provides the type of care that you need and that he or she is accepting new patients. Also, ask if they take your insurance. You have the right to choose your Doctor but Doctors also have the right to limit their practice. The variety of Physicians and the training they undergo will be discussed in a later chapter.

You have the right to access Emergency Care. This is actually a continuation of an earlier law called EMTALA. EMTALA is an acronym for Emergency Medical Treatment and Active Labor Act. This law came into existence by an act of Congress in 1986 as part of 1985 COBRA (Consolidated Omnibus Budget Reconciliation Act). *These laws can be read in their entirety on Government web page https://www.cms.gov/Regulations-and-Guidance/Legislation/EMTALA/index.html?redirect=/EMTALA/ and http://www.dol.gov/dol/topic/health-plans/cobra.htm. This law, also known as the anti-dumping law, mandates that Emergency Departments in Hospitals that are Medicare Participating (that means they can bill Medicare and includes 98% of the hospitals in the country) provide all patients that go to the ED regardless of insurance, ability to pay, race, creed, color, or national origin with a screening exam by a trained professional (either a Doctor or specially trained Nurse) to determine if they do indeed have a condition that would be considered unstable.   If they do have a medical problem that is considered unstable or if they are in active labor, they have to be treated and stabilized by that ED before they can be sent to another hospital or Doctors office.

This law came into effect when the practice of private hospitals transferring patients to county run facilities without regard for their medical condition and based solely on their financial state was rampant. People were dying. Babies were being born in parking lots. It was bad enough that congress paid attention; but only after national media started reporting on it.

The law also dictates that if a patient needs specialized medical care from another facility and they are able to treat it they have to accept that patient from the transferring facility regardless of the ability of the patient to pay. Initially, the EMTALA Act was four pages long but, like all things governmental, has grown into a huge document with very specific rules about what is and is not considered stable, at what stage of stable a patient can be transferred, and transfers for unstable patients that need specialists or admissions when the primary hospital is at capacity. All of these rules are being complicated by our litigious society where the standing laws are constantly challenged. People sue if they are not transferred to appropriate facilities and people sue if they do not like the outcomes after being transferred to an appropriate facility.

This law is also partially responsible for the over-crowding of our nation's Emergency Departments since people with no insurance know they have to be seen there even if they cannot pay for the services. People seen in the Emergency Departments are still sent a bill. This is not a free service. Nevertheless, they have to be medically treated first. It is much easier to ignore a bill for health care when you are no longer feeling ill so this practice is also a huge drain on the finances of the hospital system. In some areas, 'indigent care' is partially reimbursed through the counties but those who can't pay still show up at ED's for their care. Sad state of affairs. I hope that this is one of the areas that the progression of our national health care will address first.

The third right stated is the right to make decisions about your plan of care both before and during the treatment. You have the right to say NO to any treatment suggested even if it is not in your best interest to do so. You also have the right to understand the consequences if you do refuse treatment and, once again, options that are available to you.

There is a disclaimer on one that says this right of refusal is limited by the law and hospital policy. Basically the laws that limit this are laws of self-preservation and protection from oneself such as suicidal patients. There are also laws that protect children and elderly from decisions made by others that may not be it the patients' best interest.   These have been challenged repeatedly but so far still stand.   Hospital policy? Well, you can always ask to be transferred to a facility whose policies are more in accord with your own beliefs. Fortunately, the laws in our country still support the right of self-determination that means every person, unless confused, has the right to say what happens to them. It is a precious freedom even if health care professionals sometimes find it frustrating when trying to protect persons who make less than wise choices.

That said, what questions should you ask about your medical care so that you can make an informed decision? That of course depends on the disease process and the course of action the treatment is taking but you should ask the following questions.

*What is the disease process? That means what is the disease or injury doing to your body that makes medical intervention necessary. This part can be scary. It is never pleasant to hear that your body is not working right. Having this information is going to be very important for your next question.

*What is the treatment for what is wrong? Ask for specifics even if it sounds scary. Doctors and Nurses have to tell you all of truth if you ask for it including weird side effects that only happen to one in a million people. Do not just hear the bad scary parts. Listen to all of it. The people caring for you want to make you better almost as much as you want to be better.

*What are the side effects of the treatment? Once again, ask specific questions, even if the answers are scary. Ask percentages of patients affected by the bad side effects. This is important as, even though you may end up being the one in 1,000 who has a side effect, it is somewhat comforting to know the odds are on your side.

*What risks are involved? (See above)

*How long is it going to take to recover? Please bear in mind when you receive the response to this question that Doctors and Nurses are not fortunetellers. Every body is different and responds differently to treatments that it is subjected to. Just as some people hardly feel the effects of a common cold and some people are in bed for weeks with the same virus. There is no way that anyone can tell you exactly how your body is going to react, they can only give you a general idea about how long it takes 'most' people your age and general health to recover.

*What are the alternatives to the treatment being suggested by your Doctor? Listen carefully to this. There are almost always alternatives. If you are feeling anxious, write it down so that you can think about what the Doctor or nurse is saying later. Your advocate will come in handy here as they can help you remember and sort out all this information later. The internet is a wonderful place to do research on medical complaints BUT make sure you only use professional websites. There are still a lot of snake oil salesmen out there willing to sell you cures for anything that ails you. Don't fall for that no matter how afraid you are. You need facts in order to make an educated decision. Your physician will, of course, push for the course of action that he or she feels is in your best interest so if you have a good relationship with your Doctor, ask his opinion.

The next right listed is the right to considerate and respectful care. This is also the right most frequently violated by tired and overworked staff. Through the years I have watched many a good nurse or Doctor speak to the patient they are addressing as if the patient was mentally challenged. That is not respectful and it is certainly not considerate to the wellbeing of the patient. Most patients will not speak up and stop staff at this point either because they are intimidated by the system itself or they simply don't want to rock the boat. If a professional caregiver is speaking to you in a manner that you find disrespectful, speak up. If you have a tech that is transporting you on a gurney with no blanket and the wind has blown your gown up around your ears, stop them and tell them you want a blanket. I guarantee that most caregivers do not realize that they are being inconsiderate. They are just in a hurry to get the job done. This also encompasses the special needs of patients as far as cultural and religious needs. You have a right to have your religious items with you if they comfort you, and as long as they don't compromise your care, whether that is a cross for the wall, a prayer rug, or the wing of an eagle.

You also have the right to know who those people in your room are and what their level of training is. All hospital employees are required to wear Identification these days but if that badge is flipped around backwards, do not be afraid to ask. You have a right to know if that is a student nurse or an intern that is working on you and to decide if you are willing to let someone learn on you. Students in hospitals are well supervised and usually more than happy to do a little extra for you as they don't have that burn out mode going yet. But, you have the right to know and if you are uncomfortable with the situation ask for someone you are more comfortable with. I will address training levels of different staff in a separate chapter.

Privacy is a guaranteed right. You have the right to keep your medical history private. It cannot be discussed in the lobby, the elevator, or in the hallway outside of your room. If you have visitors, your caregivers should ask them to leave the room prior to discussing your healthcare with you unless you wish them to stay. All physical examinations are to be conducted in private. Having your gown flipped up over your head so your physician can look at your incision while your priest is in the room is not acceptable. They should ask visitors to step out of the room first. Including visitors for your roommate if you are in a shared room. Treatments also should be conducted in a private setting. Most new hospitals are going to private rooms in order to accommodate this requirement. Nevertheless, if you have a nosy roommate or it is someone you know you can ask not to have your care discussed within hearing of that person. Do not be shy about this. You are the only one who should be sharing your private information outside of the medical setting.

Paperwork is part of this privacy guarantee. Your medical records are guaranteed to be kept private. This one has caused some problems over the past few years as hospitals struggle to find the legality of who can have access to your documents. Usually you will be asked to sign a release form before records are released to anyone not directly involved in your care. The hospital is required to emphasize your privacy rights when they share information with outside parties that do have a right to know, such as your insurance company. The exceptions to this are conditions that are reportable to the public health department and abuse cases. Hospitals and caregivers are required by law to report these conditions, or suspicions of them, to the appropriate organizations.

Financial implications are also within your right to know. To be quite honest here there is a very good chance that neither your Doctor or your nurse is going to know much about the costs of specific treatments but they can direct you to the services of a social worker who can work through financial decisions with you. Be aware that hospitals have a daily charge but it varies greatly in what type of bed you are assigned. ICU is quite a lot more expensive than a Medical/Surgical bed because it requires more people hours and specialized equipment to keep you going. Moreover, there are charges for the extras although usually the basics, like your bedpan, are included in the daily charge. Hospital charges vary widely with some surprising fluctuations. For instance there is a county hospital in our area that charges substantially more than the private hospitals because private insurance charges are adjusted to compensate for the volume of uninsured (and thus high percentage of no pay) patients they see.

Another one of your rights is one that you should have addressed before you came into the hospital. You have the right to have a power of attorney. If you do not have one on admission, the hospital can provide you with a generic one and usually has a notary on staff for patient convenience. The hospital will ask if you have a power of attorney on admission. I will discuss this more in the chapter on paperwork as this is a very important document, one you do not want to be without.

You have the right to see and review your medical records. Hospitals absolutely hate it when this happens. Some have policies that require the patient to go to the medical records division on discharge and sign additional papers before seeing their records. This will change when the new healthcare act is fully implemented as it contains requirements that allow you to review your records on line. Quite a few hospitals, as of this writing, have already designed computer programs that make their records accessible to patients and patients physicians that are outside their area. They work quite well and are huge time savers for both patients and Doctors alike. Most of these are very user friendly.

Also on the list is a patient's right to expect that a hospital will take into consideration a patients specific requests for appropriate and medically indicted care and services. That means if you find some miracle cure during all of your internet research and you would like your hospital to provide that treatment for you they, at the very least, have to investigate the treatment. This does not mean they have to provide it. It means they have the responsibility to <u>consider</u> your request. The hospital also has the responsibility to arrange to transfer you to another facility if they cannot provide the requested care.

You have the right to know of any business relationships that exist between healthcare providers, educational facilities, or payers that may or may not influence the path your care follows. Known as the Stark Act after the sponsor of the Omnibus Budget Reconciliation Act of 1989; this acts as an impediment to hospitals or doctors using the system for financial gain at the expense of their patients. In other words, if your Doctor owns stock in the hospital he has to tell you that before he admits you to that hospital. It also means that if the hospital is getting a grant for providing specific treatments to patients, they have to tell you. There is another law known as the Sunshine Act that requires drug companies to report payments and gifts made to Doctors and Teaching hospitals. All this to keep everyone honest and control the conflict of interest that may not be beneficial to the patient.

If your hospital is part of a research or educational facility, they must give you the right to decline to participate in any research projects or human experimentation. This one sounds really scary but addresses legitimate concerns from earlier episodes in the evolution of healthcare when patients were experimented on without their knowledge. Think about the movie "One flew over the Cuckoo's Nest." That type of stuff really did happen. Currently "experimentation", in most cases, means something as simple as having a few extra vials of blood or other tissue taken for examination by researchers. Do not automatically reject this. If it is not going to involve pain or risk on your part, it is probably a good idea to go ahead and participate. This is how medicine advances.

You have the right to expect continuity of care. That simply means that you will not be discharged home or to another facility without the hospital arranging for your care to continue whether that be making sure your Doctor has access to your records so he can treat you at home or making contact with agencies who can provide needed medical equipment for your home use. Often times physicians request that a Home Health Care nurse visit you at home after your discharge to make sure you are doing OK. This safeguard is being used more and more frequently as patients are discharged earlier in their recovery. They will also make sure that you have a ride home or arrange for an ambulance to take you to another hospital. In addition, that you will have access to any equipment you need to facilitate your recovery at home.

One of the rights guarantees that the hospital will make available to you their policies, practices, and responsibilities. These should be reviewed if you are being admitted to a hospital for a treatment that could generate religious or moralistic debate. If the hospital policy differs from what you believe is right, choose a different hospital. If you have a complaint, the hospital has to tell you how to address it through their sometimes confusing array of administrators that handle grievances. Good hospitals want to make their patients happy. You are the customer they depend on for their continued existence as a business. If you are unhappy, tell someone. You are paying for the services. It is your right to complain and their responsibility to attempt to find a resolution to your problem that is acceptable to both parties. That includes the physicians that work in the hospital or have practice rights at that facility. Ethics committees are part of every functioning hospital.

The list of patients' rights go on to explain that in addition to the responsibilities of the hospitals, you, the patient also have reciprocal responsibility to be honest with your Doctor and Nurses about your medical history, medications you are taking, and any other health care matters that could affect the outcome to your treatment by them. You are expected to work with them to find a solution to your health care problems. Since that is the goal of anyone with a medical problem that needs hospitalization, it should be easy for you to comply. You are also expected to make 'reasonable accommodations' to staff and other patients and to comply with their rules. I will be very honest with you here and tell you that not even the staff in most hospitals know all the rules. If you are told by staff that the hospital has a rule that makes you uncomfortable or seems unlikely, ask to speak to the supervisor. The reasonable accommodations to staff and other patients basically means they can ask your 15 concerned family members to step out of the room if your roommates Doctor wants to address them privately.

The patients right acts are continuing to evolve along with the health care system. Hospitals cannot deprive you of your human rights or the rights guaranteed to you as a citizen of this country. Respect is the key element in all of this. If you feel that you are not being treated with the respect you deserve or that your patient rights are being neglected it is your responsibility to tell someone. Getting you well and out of the hospital is a team effort. It is very true that the base of the power lies with the caregivers when you are feeling less than perfect and are in foreign territory but the responsibility for defending your humanity, as always, lies with you. This is another area where having your own advocate with you can be priceless.

THE PATIENT ADVOCATE

A primary consideration for any hospital stay is to never go into a hospital by yourself if it can at all be avoided. Remember that going into a hospital means that you are not functioning at your optimum level. Hospitalization means you are either sick going in or going in to have something done to you that will probably make you feel sick for a while. Illness, lack of sleep, medications, the stress of being ill, depression, lack of routine, and the 24-hour rhythm of a hospital can make understanding simple things challenging for anyone. Hospitals and the processes that take place in them are a long way from simple. Because you will not be functioning mentally at optimal level and because the stakes are so high (your life) you should always try have an advocate with you to speak for you, to assist with simple chores, and to watch out for your safety. If you cannot have someone there 24 hours a day, at least try to have someone with you during the daylight hours when Doctors visit, tests are drawn, and drugs are given. The reasons for this will become obvious as we move through the book.

First, I have to point out that the right to have an advocate with you at all times is not one of the rights guaranteed to you as a patient in the patients' Bill of rights. As a professional caregiver, the wife of a patient, and a patient myself I personally feel it should be a guaranteed right but then I am not a congressional representative or a senator. In other countries families are encouraged to stay with their family members and to assist with their care. Our country has developed a system where efficiency denies some of the most simple of human comforts such as home cooked food or family to help you. Therefore, the hospital has the right to restrict visiting hours although most hospitals will allow you to have an advocate with you. You, as the consumer, have the right to request this. You also have the power to move your business to another facility if the hospital you are in unfairly restricts your access to an advocate.

What is an Advocate? A patient advocate is a person who watches out for you while you are too sick or too stressed to make decisions on your own. Usually a spouse, family member, or a close friend, they can help you with simple chores like adjusting the position of your bed, getting to the bathroom without falling, or figuring out the TV channels on the TV. They will also be there to question the nurses and Doctors as to the procedures that are ordered and the medications that are given. Having someone there to explain to you what the nurse or Doctor said when the drugs wear off can be priceless.

I remember when I had a knee surgery. A very young and obviously new nurse who was just coming on shift in the recovery room ordered my husband, a physician, from the room prior to giving me discharge instructions. The anesthesia for the surgery had included a drug known as a hypnotic, which, basically, erases your memory of the event. I had NO idea what I was supposed to do when we got home. Do I walk on it today? When can I take the pain pills? What did they do exactly? If my husband had not been a physician, I would have been lost. If I ever find myself in that position again I will refuse to allow my support person to be ordered from the room.

What?!?! You say. Can you do that? Remember, the practice of medicine is a business. You as the consumer have the right to demand fair treatment and good return on the money you are spending. You are also guaranteed by federal law the right to understand what is being done to you and why. If you have been given medications that make it impossible for you to understand what is being done to you, you DO have the right to have an advocate present when your care is discussed. If you do not like the way you are being treated, complain to someone. Hospitals do not want to lose your business.

The advocate, or support person if you prefer that term, that stays with you should be someone who is willing to help care for you while you are ill. Yes, you are paying the hospital to take care of you but you must understand that the hospital and the people who work there are interested in your medical condition and care. Their focus is going to be on taking vital signs, giving medications, making sure tests are done in a timely manner, and documenting the progress or lack of progress you make in your physical recovery. Helping you with the TV remote, taking the little plastic protectors off the meal plates, picking up the book that you dropped for the fifth time are not their priorities. And, while they will explain things if you ask medical staff has a tendency to speak in medical language which can make it hard to understand even if you haven't had a huge dose of pain medication.

Medicine has evolved into a system that precludes comfort in an effort to expedite the medical process. Your private physician, who has followed your medical history for years, may not visit you as most hospitals now employ 24 hour a day Doctors known as "Hospitalists". These are Doctors under contract to the hospital that stay in the hospital and see all patients admitted to the floors. Medical providers care will be addressed under the chapter by that name along with descriptions of hospital chain of command, and advice on how to talk to your providers. However, you and your advocate should be aware that the Doctor who sees you once you are admitted may be no more familiar with your medical history than the Emergency Room Doctor was.

Your patient advocate should be someone who is close enough to you that you are willing to share the knowledge of your medical history. All of it; not just the pretty parts. This is incredibly important so that they will be able to question specific treatments and medications that are part of your life. Remember, the reason for having this person with you is to have someone there to be a strong support for you when you are at your weakest and most confused point.

Your ideal advocate should also be someone who can deal with "icky stuff" coming from your body. Not everyone is going to be fortunate enough to have someone who is willing to accept this part of your care. If your advocate does not have a strong stomach or medical training do not torture them by asking them to stay in the room during procedures. All hospital floors have waiting rooms and if your advocate is going to faint or get sick at the sight of blood or other body fluids, ask them to step out when that time comes. The last thing you want is for your nurse, who is already overworked, to have to haul your friend downstairs to the emergency room instead of taking care of you.

Every normal adult feels some level of embarrassment at being too weak to care for themselves or by having fluids spill from their body unannounced. Unfortunately, if you are in a hospital you probably are that sick. Pick an advocate that you are not going to feel too embarrassed in front of should you lose control of your bowels or vomit. Sound gross? It is part of being sick. Your body is going to be trying to heal itself in addition to having all kinds of substances shoved at it by the medical community in an effort to make you better. Many of those attempts at healing and medications you are given will cause negative reactions in your body like diarrhea, nausea/vomiting, and odd body odor.

Once again, the ideal advocate to have with you is someone who is willing and ABLE to stand by you while you are sick: Someone who can help you to the bathroom if allowed, wipe vomit off your chin if needed, and do it all with a smile for the harried staff.

Another aspect to consider when choosing someone to potentially serve as your patient advocate is that the person you pick should not be someone who needs large amounts of physical comfort. A person who adores camping would be a good choice as so many of the physically uncomfortable situations your advocate finds themselves in will be more tolerable if that person can think of themselves as in a camping situation. They will have to tolerate non-optimal sleeping situations, weird noises at night, less than gourmet food, restricted personal hygiene, and strange animals (well, OK nurses and aides) coming into your room at all hours.

Medical wishes in the form of a medical power of attorney should be put in writing by everyone. Not just when being admitted to a hospital but it is even more important to have one if you are being treated in a hospital. Your advocate should be aware of what your wishes for outcome are, including the extremes that you wish the Doctors to go to in preserving your life should the absolute worst scenario present itself. No, it is not comfortable to talk to people about whether or not you want someone to do CPR on you and when to stop. I have seen the closest of married couples choke up and freeze when this question is presented. It is not something that members of our society are comfortable addressing especially when you do not feel well. Your advocate should be someone you trust to follow through with your wishes whether that is what they would choose for you or not.

Not all hospitals and/or nurses are going to be happy with a patient advocate staying with the patient. A patient advocate slows things down by questioning the process. Since that very questioning is the reason I suggest that your advocate be there, this slowing down of the process is not a consideration for you. This is your life and your body. Slow them down if you need too! If you are lucky enough to score a seasoned nurse, she will welcome your advocate warmly knowing that the time consumed in answering your questions will be saved by the assistance and comfort of you, the patient. Helping with dinner service, clean-ups, and entertainment for the patient more than makes up for the time consumed by a few questions. In addition, more and more studies are showing that a happy patient, one who is loved, heals faster than someone who is lonely and sad. A good nurse will know that and welcome your support person.

Once again, Federal law does not guarantee you the right to have another person with you all the time. It does guarantee you the right to understand what is happening to you and sometimes the only way to do that is to have someone else there with you. If the hospital that you are being admitted to does not allow for that patient support person and it is not an emergency admission, go elsewhere. Hospitals are a business and they try to keep their customers happy. Patients are customers and while the balance of power in hospitals is different for other places that you give your business to, they will still adjust their services if patients demand it.

Also, be aware that not all hospitals will provide your advocate with services. That is not their chief concern nor should it be. Hospitals exist to provide medical care to sick people. The more progressive the facility you are treated at the more likely you will encounter a system designed to accommodate family members and advocates.

The more progressive medical facilities will provide cots for sleeping and "guest trays" of food for advocates. Some facilities have private showers; most do not. Your advocate will have to find alternative ways to maintain cleanliness. Once again, it depends on the progressiveness of the facility. I have worked in and stayed in facilities from both ends of the spectrum. One of the regional hospitals I worked at in the Midwest even provided RV hookups in a special area of the parking lot for families to park their RVs while they stayed with the patients. The same facility provided really nice and comfortable rollaway cots in private rooms designed for patients and families to share. It allowed for a little private time for the personal caregivers and private shower facilities. The same facility also had little kitchenettes set up, one to a floor, with microwaves, refrigerators, water heating pots, and simple supplies (tea, coffee, crackers) for families. They were maintained by the hospital for the families of patients. Needless to say the patients that stayed there were by far the happiest I have seen in my career. I would love to see a study done on recovery times in that hospital, and others like it, versus hospitals that discourage family participation.

Of course, the opposite also exists out there. There still exist facilities where family members have to go to the lobby to use a toilet or get a glass of water. While playing advocate I have also had to sleep in solid oak desk chairs, Gerry chairs (hard as rock fold out chairs to hold paraplegics), and my own fold out chair. I have never found a hospital that was unwilling to provide linen and pillows for an advocate. While I hope to avoid ever spending another night in a hospital I now stay prepared and that includes a portable cot, which I keep in my garage. It waits there to be thrown in the trunk of the car should I ever need it. I also maintain a small "hospital survival kit" ready for use. It contains things such as shampoo, towelettes, deodorant, lotion, a toothbrush, sweat pants, a tee shirt, a change of undies, socks, and a paperback book for my comfort: A wise plan for anyone with a family member with chronic health issues that can require hospitalization at a moment's notice.

Whatever you do, do not choose an advocate who will turn into someone that the nurses have to care for also. The idea is to provide support for your loved one not add more weight to the burden of your already over worked nurse. Having worked as a nurse for many years, I can assure you that they really are over worked; caring for multiple patients and delivering primary care (that means no CNA. Many hospitals have eradicated the position of Nursing assistant for cost reasons), taking Doctors orders, transporting patients around the hospital, delivering medications to patients, admissions, discharges, and documenting progress hourly on ALL of their patients. Most nurses are too busy already.

Finally, make sure your advocate knows in advance that staying with you is not going to be a vacation. They will sleep in less than desirable conditions being awakened every hour by people caring for you, eat less then desirable food, and be bored to death during the long daylight hours of watching you sleeping and endless TV reruns of Andy Griffith shows. In addition, a huge emotional element needs to be taken into account here. It is very difficult to watch someone that you care about be that sick. Being an advocate is physically and emotionally draining. Make sure that you explain that to your advocate beforehand. You should feel very grateful that you are loved to this degree.

What, you ask, am I to do if I don't have someone willing to serve as my patient advocate? The answer is that most people that go into a hospital do not have a personal advocate. Try to have someone at least stay with you during the hours when the Doctors do rounds so they can ask questions you may not think of or are too confused to ask and remind you later what the Doctor said. A family member, close friend, or even your religious leader can fill this roll.

You can also sign privacy wavers, which will allow the nurse caring for you to answer questions over the phone to one family member. Please, do not expect the nurse to talk to everyone in your family. Choose one person you trust who can keep the rest of your family and friends advised. Many hospitals now ask you on admission for a family advocate name and number. This one person will be kept abreast of your condition and other family members can call that person for updates instead of flooding the hospital switchboard with calls. This person can also serve as a telephone advocate if they are unable to stay with you. It is possible to have them on speaker phone while the Doctor speaks with you.

Some hospitals still employ professional patient advocates who can help you understand what is being done for you and to you. They can also address medication questions with pharmacists and review tests with you. They are NOT available to assist with your comfort or entertainment. And they are not allowed legally to advice you about your care, only to help you understand it. Most hospitals have in the last few years cut this position from their rosters when looking at cost cutting measures. It was considered an unnecessary luxury to have a nurse on staff with the sole responsibility of explaining things to patients. I think that eventually the more progressive hospitals will recognize the importance of this position and again start hiring nurses to fill it.

If you have concerns and no patient advocate is available you can also ask to speak to the social worker or case manager. These people in this position are usually stretched very thin but will try their best to help you understand the care being provided. Once again, they are NOT available to help you with comfort measures.

Another option that may be open to you is the hospital chaplain. Not all chaplains feel comfortable in this roll and it is best to ask before assuming.

Provider point- It is in your best interest, as well as your patients, to welcome these family members or friends to assist in the care of your patient. Yes, having an additional person in the room can feel intimidating especially for new nurses but a good advocate can lessen your workload immensely. In addition, stop and think about how you would feel in the position of the patient. Do you want to be there all by yourself?

Please do not think of family as a hindrance. Yes, over the years I have met family members that I have had to ask to leave the room and ones that I would have liked to toss out the window. Every nurse I know has a least one horror story about a family member who called them into the room at a busy moment to ask for something not related to the patient. Not everyone is suited to the role of patient support any more than everyone is suited to being a nurse or a Doctor. If a family member is behaving inappropriately, try teaching them. Most nurses are good teachers; it's part of the nursing process. When the daughter sitting in the chair next to the sleeping mother hits the call light for the umpteenth time in the first hour to ask you to change the channel on the TV again; show her how to do it herself. Explain to them how much you appreciate them being there for your patient. Tell them, politely please, that as a patient support person it is important for them to participate. There have indeed been times I wanted to post the story of the "little boy who cried wolf" in a room without realizing that in doing so I have become the wolf.

Yes, you do have the right to gently explain to advocates that have a tendency to "ride the bell', that caring for them is not part of your work load and to remind them that they are there to care for their loved one. I have had this discussion with family members myself. There is nothing worse than a family member that hits the call button to have you drop what you are doing to 'adjust' the bed for their loved one or change the channel on the television. Teach them how to do it themselves if they don't know how. Giving patient advocates a brief verbal orientation to the room and hospital policies will save you time and energy as most really are there to help the family member or friend that they love. Handing them one of those huge packages that administration put together with all the required paperwork in it is not going to do it. Very few people even open those up. If you do not have time to explain it or you have run into one of the rare ones that thinks since their family member is paying such an outrageous bill they should benefit too, call your supervisor and let them deal with it. You, as the patients nurse, need to remain the good guy.

And family food. At least offer the family some kind of beverage, even if it's just ice water. One of the most memorable people in a hospital setting was a CNA who kept a package of breakfast hot pockets in the staff freezer for family members of patients. Turns out, she was a patient, at one point, on an Oncology floor and the family member that stayed with her didn't eat for two days. She took it upon herself to make sure that did not happen to other people's families. Do not freak out if they share with their family member unless the patient is on a very strict diet. Just document it. I mean, have you ever tasted the food you serve your patients? There is a later chapter that will address hospital food in more detail, frightening as that is.

I have also seen, very rarely, advocates that I believe were Munchausen's by proxy, a true psychological phenomenon where people seek attention for themselves by exaggerating the symptoms of the patient. If you find yourself in the rare, but possible position of having to deal with one of these people ask the social worker or your supervisor to intervene. The idea of an advocate is to assure a safe and comfortable stay for your patient not to increase your workload. Remember those shifts when you had to assist with the feeding of four of your five patients? What if even two of those patients had an advocate with them to help them eat or to hand them the urinal? Think of the time you will save. IN ADDITION, stop and think about how you will feel if you are ever in their place.

One of my primary responses to nurses complaining about a bad day they are having is, "It could always be worse. You could be lying in one of those beds being treated by a nurse who is cranky because of the quality of her day."

And finally, a note to those administrators of hospitals who discourage family interaction. Having a family member who is trained to care for your patient by a good caring nurse is going to make that patient and family happier with the hospital experience and more comfortable with the situation when they go home. The patient whose family is trained to take care of them will have a much lower rate of recidivism because they will be comfortable with the situation at home.

It is in the hospitals best interest to allow patients to have an advocate with them and in the patient's best interest to choose an advocate wisely to assist with their care. Healthcare is a team effort and family is part of that team. Patients heal faster when they have loving family caring for them and don't just sit numbly in the hospital bed waiting for the next shot or test. Any issues that arise are so much easier to deal with when the patient and the family know that you are doing everything you can do to make them healthy again.

How not to sign away your first born during Registration and admitting

The personality of a medical center is readily palpable by the greeting received walking through the front door. Some hospitals have volunteers staffing the front desk who (because they are volunteers?) are cheerful and helpful. They can bring you a wheelchair or direct you to where you are going. That initial smile can make or break a visit. One of our local hospitals recently cut back on their volunteer program with the intent that they could reduce workman's comp costs. I think the cost in happy patients is more than going to outweigh the cost of worker's comp insurance for those wonderful pink ladies. The intimidation factor of walking into a large medical facility when you are not feeling well or are going for yet another procedure, is under-estimated even for those of us that work in those facilities. If avoiding stress is primary to speed of recovery then avoiding that initial lost feeling when walking into another large facility needs to be addressed and is easily resolved by staffing the volunteer desk with volunteers. Think Walmart and Disneyland! They both know the wisdom of a greeter at the door.

The registration process is first in this field day of interaction with 'care' providers. My husband and I have sat at a desk and had a young woman completely ignore us for 10 minutes while typing into her computer. If it had been a restaurant, we would have left.

Unfortunately, in health care there is not that option. You sit and you wait. By contrast, we have also had friendly volunteer walk us over to the registration desk and introduce us to the registration clerk. What a great feeling that was! Being recognized as an individual and not just another test waiting in the lobby is invaluable.

Privacy can be paramount. I was once horrified to overhear, while waiting in a hospital lobby, a patients financial status being discussed within earshot of other patients, including income, assets, and payment options for a very private medical procedure. The patient was obviously horrified; the clerk never noticed their discomfort. With the advent of the HIPAA regulations, most hospitals now have closed in little offices for interviewing the patients for registration. These inexpensive cubicles, while for the most part are not sound proof, are definitely an improvement over the old method of public discussion of finances and reasons for health care.

The smiling or frowning face of the registration person can set the tone for the hospital stay. I give the registration clerks credit for maintaining those smiles all day long. They are in a position where they are asking insurance and financial questions from someone who probably does not feel very well and is a little cranky because of it. In addition, it takes time and the ability to distract the patient from the drawn out process. They have to verify the insurance, make all those copies, and then get you to sign them. And don't forget to initial here!

These clerks have little or no medical training so do not expect them to answer questions about your stay or procedure. They are not qualified to answer your medical questions. But then, the nurses you meet later will not be qualified to answer your paperwork questions. Neither my husband nor I had ever read any of this paperwork prior to being patients ourselves. We were amazed and, sometimes, amused by what we found in that paperwork when we started really reading it for this book.

The registration clerks, also, cannot answer your questions about the cost of your stay. However, if you are really concerned you can ask at this time to speak to a financial advisor or social worker.

So, what are you signing? The registration process depends on why and how you are being admitted to the hospital. If you are going in through the Emergency Department of a hospital there is a federal law that stops the registration clerk or anyone else from asking you for your insurance information before you are seen AND given a preliminary medical evaluation. This law is called the EMTALA law and was addressed in detail in the patient rights section. EMTALA stands for Emergency Medical Treatment and Active Labor Act. The registration process in the ED is dictated by this law and differs from the general admission process of the hospital. I will address that process in the chapter on Emergency Rooms. The paperwork you will be asked to sign is the same general paperwork addressed here.

Registration begins with a form, or set of questions if the hospital is up to date on the computer systems, that are reminiscent of a job application form. Standard stuff like name, date of birth, address, phone; they will also ask you for insurance information, employers, and close relatives. This is all information that is required by law to be kept confidential so, allowing for human error, you are safe in disclosing this information to the clerk that asks you for it.

The clerk will want copies of your insurance cards and some form of ID. The ID did not use to be a requirement until insurance fraud became rampant. Now the hospitals like to verify that they are actually billing the right insurance for the right patient. Be aware that if you are not an emergency patient and do not have insurance, private hospitals have the right to send you to a facility that is funded to help with patients who cannot pay for their own care.

Understand that every hospital has their own outline for the form they use. They will contain almost all of the information I give here; some in more flowery, confusing legalize, and others actually give it to you in English (that is refreshing). So if your forms do not follow this writing exactly, well just know that most of this stuff is probably in there somewhere.

Allowing for the variance in the type and content of paperwork, but after this initial basic information, you will be asked to read and sign a Conditions of Admission form. This includes admission for outpatient procedures like lab draws, EKG's, and x-rays too.

The Conditions of Admissions is a very long form. This is one of those forms that no one ever reads, especially when they are not feeling well, and everyone signs because they want to get on with it. So now, let us get on with the boring part of this book and let you know what it says.

This form usually starts out with a short paragraph on definitions. Things like "Hospital". Now I know you are thinking that you know what a hospital is, that is why you are sitting in front of the desk in one, and why would they feel the need to define that. The answer to that is that this form will explain to you what hospital you are at, just in case you have forgotten since you walked in the front door or missed that giant sign out front. Remember, lawyers designed these forms.

Next, it will explain to you what a patient and a patient's legal representative are. You are thinking "But I'm the patient!" Well, according to most of these forms you are not the patient until you are through the registration process, meaning after the paperwork is signed. And patients legal representative? It explains in a very long sentence, that a legal representative has to be someone named in a Power of Attorney or Advanced Directive. Some hospitals will provide you with a generic copy of an Advance Directive if you request one. I would strongly recommend that an Attorney draw up this form so there is no question as to the legitimacy of the document. You do not want anyone debating the legality of your last wishes over you while they are doing CPR or asking your long lost cousin twice removed whom you have not seen in 25 years, if he knows what your wishes would be in a case like this.

Next, the legalese will explain to you that when this document refers to 'you' it actually means You. I know, that is shocking. Who would have thought it? And that when the document refers to "We", "Us", or "our" it is talking about the hospital. "Insurance" does indeed mean insurance or other plan that will help you pay the bill. (Yes, this is all really in that paperwork.)

Last on definitions is a term called "full charges". Now this can be confusing as hospitals charge differently based on whether or not you have insurance, and whether or not the hospital has a relationship or contract with your insurance company which allows for discounts or reductions. Hospitals have room to negotiate for their costs and they will work with you on some things if you find yourself in financial need. During the registration process is not the time to do that. That needs to be done later with a social worker or one of the financial officers of the hospital. Hopefully, you have a good insurance plan that does the negotiating for you. If not, it will involve a very frustrating series of phone calls until you locate the correct person in the business office to talk too. No, I do not have suggestion to get through this part. My personal feeling on some of it is that the more difficult they make it the more likely people will not pursue those discounts.

One of the next paragraphs on this page will be the Consent to Medical and Surgical Procedures. This paragraph tells you, in generalized language, all the exciting things the hospital can do to you while you are there and then, also in generalized language, that they are not responsible for the stuff they are going to do to you. Do not worry too much about this. It is a generalized form. If the hospital causes you harm they are still responsible. This is a safe guard for them against the 'normal' side effects of some of the tests and treatments you may be subjected to. If you are being treated as an outpatient, your Doctor should have already explained the risks and benefits to you. If you are an in-patient you have the right to ask the Nurse, Doctor, or Technician what tests are being done, why they are being done, and what side effects, if any, are possible. Most of the time the benefits of an ordered test far out-weigh the risks of the same and have already been evaluated by the ordering Doctor.

Somewhere in this form, there is a Consent to Electronic Recording. This one is somewhat uncomfortable for some people as it gives the hospital the right to take pictures or films of you and use them for training purposes. Some of the forms I have seen even go so far as to state that you are giving permission to have your photo used for advertising. I cannot believe that in this day of guarded privacy, any hospital would utilize pictures of you without specific information and a second signed consent but I suppose it could happen. I think this clause is more for the generalized protection of the hospital in case they accidentally have someone showing in the background of some photo or film.

While this form may also address the notice of Privacy Protection there is usually an entirely separate pamphlet, flyer, or print out telling you about your HIPAA rights. This also includes information on your right of privacy. In 1996 this law was passed with its main purpose being to safeguard peoples insurance if they lost or changed their job but has evolved into a much more complicated state. This law now also addresses the need for electronic records to facilitate Medicare billing and patient care but it is probably best known for the privacy law that was written into it. HIPAA, which stands for Health Insurance Portability and Accountability Act, like all things created by our government in an effort to make things easier, it is huge, hard to understand, and complicated. Like all government works, after they finished complicating the law they started writing the volumes needed to explain this one too. If you are interested in reading it, you can find the law and all its required explanations at www.hhs.gov , which is the web site for the United States Department of Health and Human Resources. You can always print out a copy and take it with you in case you have trouble getting to sleep while you are in the hospital.

Most hospitals, with Doctors permission, will allow you to hire a private duty nurse to help take care of you while you are in their facility. The nurses that the hospital pays to be on staff are, for the most part, general care nurses and have four or 5 patients to take care of everyday. If you feel that you will need more care than those quotas will allow, you have the option, at your own expense and with the Doctors (the one providing primary care in the hospital) permission, to hire a private care nurse. I have personally served in this role to a family member providing involved care in a hospital I was not employed at. The house nurses' were very happy to have me there as it lightened their load considerably and the Doctor was happy that his patient had one on one care. This is also an option if you don't have a friend or family member willing to serve as your advocate and you can afford it. Be aware hiring a private duty Nurse is a very expensive proposition and does require a Doctors written order to alleviate hospital legal concerns.

There is also a paragraph, somewhere in this form, that protects students in training. It advises you, the patient, that some of the people who treat you may be in the process of learning to provide care to patients. Not to worry. Most students will identify themselves as such before they touch you. All nurses and Doctors are required to do some hospital time as part of their training. Senior personnel supervise them during this training. If you are shy of having a trainee practice or learn on you, tell them. Sometimes the students are the better caregivers as they are fresh and new, are trying very hard to learn, and trying to impress their instructors.

This is also the form that will advise you that the Doctors do not work for the hospital. Surprised? Not even the Doctors who work on the floors of the hospital actually work for the hospital itself although there are exceptions to every rule. They are usually employees of a group of physicians that have a contract with the hospital to provide services there. It is a long held misconception that the Doctors run the hospital. Administrators run hospitals. Doctors sign contracts with administrators so they have somewhere to put their sick patients and access to the large expensive machines that do the tests to tell them what is wrong with their patients. There are governing boards for the Doctors that are contracted there and if you ever have an issue with a Doctor, tell the hospital representative and they will address it with the Doctors who make up this board.

Some hospitals allow physicians to own stock in their hospitals. That brings us to the disclosure law. This is the law, known as the Stark

Act, which dictates that if a Doctor owns interest in a hospital or clinic or testing facility, they must disclose to their patients that they may profit from an admission or ordered tests. The law was put into place to safeguard patients from unscrupulous physicians ordering unnecessary tests or admissions in order to make money and was discussed in the chapter on patient's rights.

Also, be aware that Doctors bill separately from the hospital. The Doctors charges for care are not included in the bill that the hospital compiles. You will get a separate bill from the Group that your physician works for. In fact, every Doctor who has anything to do with your care while you are in the hospital will send you or your insurance a bill. This includes the ones that you never see; the radiologist, pathologist, anesthesiologist, and other specialists your primary Doctor consults. One of the later chapters will address the array of people, including Doctors that may have something to do with your care. Doctors, too, have some flexibility with their charges but be aware that these are separate.

Speaking of bills, this form will probably also contain Financial Agreements. It will tell you that they, the hospital, will bill your insurance and that you agree to pay whatever the insurance does not pay; co-pays, deductibles, etc. It will warn you that your insurance may refuse to pay. That is a scary thought but sometimes true. Insurance companies are notorious for refusing payment based on services that are not covered by your plan, or the hospital is not in the insurance company's network, or that they wanted to you to have authorization before you had something done, or because the insurance company does not think what you had done was necessary. Most often, when the insurance company refuses to pay, if you challenge them they will respond positively. They do not really expect you to let them know in advance if you are planning on breaking your leg or having a heart attack. There are also federal and state level insurance regulatory organizations you can appeal to if you have this problem. However, most hospitals and Doctors will make sure that things are documented in such a way that the insurance will pay. (Their paycheck depends on it.) Part of this agreement is that you are giving the hospital permission to challenge the insurance company for anything they refuse to pay on, so that is a positive. They want to be paid as much as you want them to be paid.

Prior authorization is on the upswing as hospitals and Doctors do not like fighting for their money any more then you do. Prior authorization just means that the hospital will call the insurance company and get a guarantee that they will be paid before they perform any tests. In addition, unless your Doctor is really out there, he is not going to order a test that is not medically necessary.

There will probably also be a paragraph advising you that if you do not have insurance you will be financially responsible for the total cost incurred. However, as I said earlier, the hospital will also work with you including discounts and helping you find government or outside financial assistance.   This should not be a problem if you have followed the law that now mandates that you have insurance but there are always exceptions.

Credit checks are sometimes written in here although I am not sure why. Financing a hospital stay is not usually in the cards for patients and I have never heard of a patient being refused services because they had a less then desirable credit score. I have heard financial representatives of a hospital call a county run facility and assist a patient in arranging to have their elective surgery done there instead of at the private facility. The frightening part of that was that the county run facility was charging almost 1/3 more for the same service as the private hospital and the patient was going to get that bill. Sometimes it just does not make sense.

These forms contain third party liability agreements. This sounds confusing but is not really. It means that if someone else has caused your hospitalization (think car accident) because of the injury caused to you by their actions, they are financially responsible for treatment that injury requires; the hospital can go after them for any additional cost incurred. That means they have the right to make the person that injured you pay your deductible and any percentages not covered by your insurance plan. Or, if you have no insurance, the hospital has the right to sue that person for the costs of your stay. In fact, if a lawsuit ensues because of the accident you can expect to have to sign a release of payment for the medical costs incurred to the lawyer handling your case.

There are usually two separate paragraphs in this form about property. One will address medical property used in services. Basically, if you buy it, it is yours. So you can take your bedpan home with you along with the flimsy little water pitcher. There is other equipment (some of it actually useful) also included in this but if you have a question about what you can take with you when you leave, ask. The nurses will tell you. Some equipment is considered as a rental from the hospital and you cannot maintain possession of that. Believe it or not I once had to help track down a very expensive portable ventilator that a patient took home with them thinking that if they had used it, it was theirs. Not so!

The second paragraph on property will address what you should and should not bring into the hospital with you. Generally, do not take anything into the hospital with you that you are willing to risk losing. The hospital will not be responsible for your personal property and they cannot safe guard your possessions while you are there. If for instance, you take your laptop with you. Do you have a support person or an advocate staying with you who can watch it while you are getting your x-rays? If not, best to leave it home. Hospitals all have safes where they can lock up your wallet for you during your stay. You will not have access to it during your stay as it goes through a safe guarding procedure before being locked up, but it will be safe until you are released to go home. Thefts are notorious in hospital settings. People steal from each other and from the hospital so consider yourself forewarned.

Last, but not least is the Patient certification; the long awaited, magic part that allows you finally to become the patient. This is the part of the form where you sign to verify that you did indeed read and understand all of the above. Since you probably did not read any of it including the part where you sign that you did read it, well, it all goes back to that infamous catch 22.

The Conditions of Admissions may or may not contain more or less information than what I have included here. This is a generalization of several forms I have read over the course of many years. Once again, every hospital has its own form unless it is part of one of the giant conglomerate systems. In that case, it will be different from the forms of all the other giant conglomerate hospital systems. That also goes for the other forms you will receive. A few are routine as the understanding of the material in them is federal law. For instance, the afore mentioned HIPAA law is usually explained in a hand out to the patient as is the EMTALA law. There may be a handout that explains the paperwork you have already signed such as patient rights.

Some hospitals have handouts on how to get assistance in the hospital if you are displeased with the service or have a complaint. Some hospitals have what they call rapid response teams (A rapid response team is someone to call if you think you are sicker than you should be and wish to be re-evaluated) and they will give you a pamphlet explaining what that is and how to implement it. The variety of paperwork is endless and, quite honestly, mind numbing. You can always save it in your hospital night stand for those nights when you can't sleep. Hospital paperwork is one of the best sleep aids hospitals provide.

The diversity of the paperwork that hospitals hand out is as diverse as the hospitals that create them. Very few people take the time to read it all or try to understand it. They trust the system to tell them where to sign and initial. It is honest caring people that run these facilities and that have designed the paperwork for your stay. It is honest and caring people that will tell you where to sign and initial. It is your responsibility to work with them. If you want to know what you are signing, ask. Someone will tell you.

"I would have gone to the clinic but the game went into overtime" Or Welcome to the Emergency Department

While not all admissions to a hospital come through the Emergency Department, a large percentage do. Even patients that have personal, caring physicians can find themselves in the Emergency Department line-up if they get sick on a weekend or at night. And federal statistics show that 40% of patients treated in the emergency room will end up admitted to the floor. Unfortunately, for patients, more and more physicians are refusing to take call when there is a hospitalist on duty at the local facility. While I completely understand the need to have a private life and the desire to not be disturbed at all hours of the day and night, I also find the depersonalization of medical care to be very frightening. Having a physician who knows your medical and personal history and is willing to be called on weekends or at night is rapidly becoming a luxury. If you are one of the lucky few who still has such a Doctor, take good care of him or her! For the rest of you there is... (Imagine dramatic music here) the Emergency Room.

For starters, the Emergency Room is no longer called Emergency Room. The correct term is Emergency Department and while the art of emergency medicine has evolved along with the phraseology that describes the place itself, it is still one of the least respected places in the modern hospital. To fully understand the lack of respect you need to realize that most Doctors and Nurses have a tendency toward being obsessive/compulsive. They like order. Everything needs to be in its place and at the proper time. Emergency rooms are superficially organized chaos. There is no other way to describe them. Attempts have been made in recent years to better control the functioning of this department: Specific areas are assigned to specific duties (i.e. pediatrics) with specially trained personnel and specialized equipment. Some ED's are even advertising call lines where you can call in and schedule a time to have your emergency. It's all done with the positive thought bringing that aforementioned organization to a reality. It's a nice idea and it works very well until, well, until a true emergency happens. Then, while the specialized people all function within their specialty, your reserved time-frame is completely lost.

Most people don't have a true appreciation for the chaos that can ensue in these places. I am reminded of a day in the critical care area of a large Northern California Emergency room. It had been a slow day. Nothing critical; no heart attacks, strokes, or major trauma had come in. Because of that we were treating patients in the critical area that would have been better suited to a clinic because the "rapid care" area of the ED was packed. (Rapid care area is the term used to describe the area used to treat clinic type patients.) And it was flu season so we were inundated with patients complaining of coughs, sniffles, nausea, and generalized aches and pains. Like most people that don't feel well, these people were getting cranky that they had to wait, although the wait times were fairly short as these things go. Then it happened. First the car accident with 5 patients including two critical children, came in. Next the stroke patient with full right sided paralysis. Then an ambulance arrived with a patient who was having trouble breathing. His heart stopped as they came through the doors. All of these patients within 15 minutes of each other. We were sending technicians to the radiology department for gurneys because all of our critical beds were full. The non-critical patients were being pushed on their gurneys into the hallway to accommodate the patients that were going to die without immediate care. I was assisting with the patient whose heart had stopped when the curtain separating the beds was thrown open by an angry middle aged woman who began shouting that it was her turn to be seen by the Doctor and she was not going into the hallway when the patient we were working on had jumped the line. The Doctor giving the orders and trying to save the poor man's life froze. You could see the flush of anger crawl up his neckline and into his face. He turned to her slowly and in a voice that was cold as ice told her, "This is an emergency room. We treat emergencies first. If you would like all of the attention that this 'line jumper' is getting just sit back down in that bed and die. As soon as your heart stops we will all rush in and give you the attention you seem to so desperately want." The woman's mouth moved without sound for several seconds as she stared at the Doctor. She surveyed the room with the tubes, IV's, radiology equipment, and the tech doing hard compressions on the dying man's chest; you could see her absorbing the sounds and the smells of death. Then she turned and walked out the doors of the ED. The clerks told us later that she kept on walking in that hospital gown until she was out the front door.

The point being that if you are going to be seen in an emergency department you need to understand that the people that work there are trained to work on a triage system. Triage is a French word meaning 'to sort' and in an emergency department that means sorted, and treated, in the order of severity of injury or illness. If you are not the sickest one in the place you are not going to get treated first, unless of course, you become the sickest person.

The triage process in an Emergency Department begins when you walk up to the registration desk. If you are having chest pain, shortness of breath, severe pain, or are gushing blood; tell them. Give them your name and then tell them what is wrong if it is something that you feel is life threatening. Do not insist on telling the registration clerk what is wrong with you if the reason you are here is not life threatening. They will ask you that in the "triage room". Also, do not lie about having one of these symptoms just to get in faster. That might get you into the triage room faster but it will also earn you a full work up and probably a 23-hour hold upstairs.

The emergency department of most hospitals have become inundated with scores of people who don't have primary care providers either by choice or from lack of monetary means. After 25 years of treating patients in "emergency situations" I still feel as though most of the patients that come to an emergency room truly believe they have an emergency. I completely understand the frustration of personnel specifically trained in emergency medicine when they are presented, at 3 o clock in the morning, with a sprained ankle that happened 4 weeks ago or an otherwise healthy 20 year old that threw up once 8 hours ago and wants to make sure it won't happen again since it was unpleasant. It is, for most of us, very difficult to perceive that these people truly feel they have an emergency. Unfortunately, the frequent callous reception of patients presenting with less than emergent complaints can show. It also has a tendency to harden the perceptive abilities of otherwise caring individuals. Great care and training needs to be given to the choice of triage nurses who do the initial evaluation of presenting patients. Experience is priceless in these areas as years of interpreting physical presentation can be a great asset in determining the truly emergent patients.

So what can you expect in the Emergency department? It varies greatly and fluctuates with the area you live in, seasons, time of day, and day of the week. Anymore, you should expect to wait. Bring a good book with you. As I already stated, modern hospitals are badly overcrowded. Patients with no insurance who know they cannot be turned away, patients with no primary care Doctor to call because normally they feel fine, people who don't want to wait a week to see their own Doctor, transfers in from other hospitals that are waiting for a bed upstairs, and people who really do have a real emergency. All of these people are in the waiting room with you waiting to be seen.

There are two ways to get to an Emergency Department; walking in the lobby doors or by ambulance. If you are a walk-in patient the first thing you will do is sign in at the registration desk. As I said earlier this is just simple information time, guarded by the EMTALA laws. Your name, date of birth, and address may be asked although one of the hospitals I worked in had to stop asking for addresses as they served a large population of homeless people and someone complained that the address question was discriminatory.

As I said earlier, the Person who does the preliminary registration will probably ask you if you are short of breath, are bleeding, or are having chest pains. This person is not trained in medicine so don't go into detail. The question is there to help start the triage process. If you have one of these complaints one of the nurses will be notified immediately and unless the ED is inundated (a not uncommon condition these days) that nurse will be out to assess you soon.

Whether you have to wait for a while or are seen immediately, the next step is the triage room. This is a room equipped with equipment to take basic vital signs. One Registered nurse or intermediate provider like a Physician's Assistant usually mans it. Rarely, you will find a Doctor doing triage although this trend is growing as the possibilities of litigation increase with the over-crowding. Whoever greets you into the room will take your blood pressure, heart rate, respiratory rate, oxygen saturation level, temperature, and ask you if to rate your pain level. They will weigh you and ask for your height. Those are the basic vital signs. You will be asked why you are in the Emergency Department. Answer truthfully. The outline for your treatment will be designed around what you tell the triage person.

When you are asked if you have any medical problems now or in the past please bear in mind that this is a simple triage process. The Triage person does not want to know that you had a very difficult time when they took your tonsils out at age 8. You will, depending on your complaint, either be asked to sit and wait or, if you have specific complaints that can be symptoms of life threatening conditions (i.e. Chest pains, shortness of breath, profound bleeding) the triage process will be more involved.

If it is determined that you are suffering from a life threatening condition, you should be taken into a room in the back right away. If your complaint is less threatening, you will be asked a series of other questions that will explore your complaint further and help staff decide where to put you in the line-up of patients who are waiting.

When did your complaint start? This is important for determining the possible severity of your condition. Someone who has been throwing up and had diarrhea for 4 days will probably be sicker than someone who threw up once this morning after they ate the sausage that tasted funny or upon waking up with a mind blowing hang-over. The human body will deal with illness on its own for quite a while before it starts to tire out. Once again, don't exaggerate. Professional providers are usually very good at reading body language and if they feel you are not 100% truthful or overly dramatic they can be less then receptive.

You will be asked if you have ever had these symptoms before. This is also important in helping these providers determine the triage category you fit into. If you have had the same problem every two weeks for the past 6 months, the symptoms have not changed in that time, and you are still alive, you are not considered a high-level triage. Don't despair. This is not a game show. You will get treated just not necessarily before the guy that came in behind you that just turned blue and passed out.

Your triage person will ask you to rate the pain. Most pain scales are designed on a 1 to 10 scale with 1 being no pain at all, and 10 being the worst pain you have ever had in your life. Some hospitals are now using the 1 to 5 pain scale. Same difference. Don't exaggerate here. If you've been blessed to never have had any pain in your life and now you have sprained your ankle, it is probably not a good idea to tell the nurse that your pain is a 10, even if to you it is the worst pain you have ever had. You may be shown a little chart with a series of faces correlating with the numbers on the pain scale. 0 is a smiling face; 10 is a face obviously in agony with tears flowing down its cheeks. The numbers in between are all variations of pain. It looks a little silly but if you are one of the few blessed out there who has never had pain before this can help you reasonably evaluate yourself.

Pain is considered the fifth vital sign. Hospital personal are taught not to doubt a patient's pain level: to take the patient at their word. Unfortunately, emergency room workers can, and frequently do, develop a tendency to disbelieve patients when it comes to pain evaluation. I am not sure why this happens. Perhaps it has to do with the, all too human, need to help and the frustration at not always being able too. It is also probably also due to the number of people who do exaggerate their pain levels. Compassion overload is a very real occurrence among long term emergency workers.

There is also the factor of drug abusers who misuse emergency rooms to feed their habit. Vicodin, Percocet, and some of the other opiates that are prescribed for pain, are addictive. It is, unfortunately, quite common for people who cannot get their own physicians to prescribe the quantity of pain medications that they require to go to various ED's in order to feed their habit. I have had calls from two surrounding hospitals within a few hours of each other asking about the same patient that we had just sent out with a prescription for one of these drugs. He had shown up at both of their facilities with the same complaint that he presented at our ED. He was well known to both of those hospitals and when they refused to give him the drugs he requested, he found another hospital. While prescription abusers are a small percentage of the population they do cause problems as they 'harden' the emergency care providers to real pain.

Prescription Narcotics have an extraordinarily huge mark-up when they are sold on the street. Many heroin addicts will point to a predisposing addiction to prescription pain medications that cost more than they could afford and their path to a more affordable alternative. Once again this speaks to the addictive properties of these drugs. There have been many attempts at trying to control the seemingly indiscriminant prescribing of these drugs through emergency departments. There is even a federally funded phone line that physicians can call to check and see when and how much of these drugs have been prescribed to the patient that they are currently seeing. While I think that controlling these drugs is important I also feel that the focus on the dispensing through ED's is creating a problem with compassion towards patients that really need these drugs. I do not believe it is in the patients best interest for a physician who has seen them once, to decide if they are really in pain or not. Limited numbers of pills and a referral to the clinic or back to the patient's primary care physician could solve this without risking not treating a patient who is really in pain.

Chronic pain is the issue. Normally when you begin to feel pain your sympathetic nervous system kicks in and your body attempts to compensate. Your heart rate goes up, your blood pressure rises, and you breathe faster. People with chronic pain lose these compensatory fluctuations in their vital signs even when they are in excruciating pain. Since most triage providers base their assessments on the presented vital signs in conjuncture with the patients complaint this can create a problem. I once took a family member who was in excruciating pain to the ED with the flair up of a chronic condition. This person is normally very stoic and yet when the triage person asked the pain level he gave them a 10 in reply. His pain was a 10! The condition he suffered from had a primary presentation of pain as the initial symptom. He has an extensive medical history and does not present with an elevated heart rate or blood pressure. When he said "10" I saw the PA roll his eyes and knew we were in trouble. We were returned to the lobby and by the time he was treated in the back he was so severely ill that he had to be admitted to ICU and was in the hospital for almost two weeks. All because someone who had never met him before assumed he was exaggerating his pain. Had he been treated immediately the condition could have been controlled early and not progressed to a critical care level.

Pain is subjective. People have different tolerance levels for pain. Just because one person can tolerate the pain being experienced with an application of an ice pack does not mean that the next person will not require an IV and strong IV pain medications to control it. Our bodies are all very unique and that needs to be respected by the care givers. All too frequently it is not.

So what to do if you encounter someone who is not taking your complaint as seriously as you perceive it to be? First of all, ask to be re-triaged. In most cases this will not be met kindly. No one likes to admit they are wrong. If that request does not work you can ask to speak to a supervisor. ED supervisors are trained in triage and are usually more experienced than the triage person. If that is refused you can ask to speak to the house supervisor. Be warned that not all Nursing Supervisors are trained in Emergency medicine. That is a specialty; but they are trained in keeping the customer (that's you) happy. At the very least you will have an explanation as to why you are having to wait so long. Don't be rude or caustic with the staff. They are just doing a job. Worst case scenario you may have to go to a different ED. The hospital may really be too busy to get to you even if you are as sick as you think you are. As in the above scenario, it happens. There is no predicting when an emergency is going to happen. I have seen codes worked in the hallway because the ED was overwhelmed. Even though you are feeling sick enough that you have taken yourself to the ED, try to be fair in your evaluation and trust of the staff. Most of them are very good and caring people. Yes, they are overwhelmed and burn-out is a real phenomenon but most of the providers got into that career and kept at it because they like people.

So why don't I just take an ambulance to the hospital? They get in right away. This is one of the most misleading and system abusing beliefs out there. Ambulances do go in the back door and straight into the ED but the patients that are transported by ambulance are still subject to the triage system. When you call an ambulance you are examined by the paramedic prior to transport. If you have called the ambulance to avoid a wait time, chances are the Paramedic will tell the hospital that when they call in on the radio to let the hospital know you are coming. This can land you in the bad graces of the staff in the ED before you even get there. Like I said, you will still be subject to the hospital triage system and sent to the lobby if you are not the sickest of the lot. No one likes someone who abuses the system. Back in the days when I worked on an ambulance I once transported a patient who had (I kid you not) fingertip pain. Just one finger! No swelling, no redness, just the tip of one finger hurt and she didn't want to have to wait to have it looked at. The law in California made it mandatory that we transport her by ambulance because she had requested it. All of the hospitals in town were incredibly busy that day. When I called it in on the radio I was met with a long pause before the radio nurse came back and told us that the patient would be going to the lobby for a "therapeutic wait." I'm not sure how long that wait ended up being but from the anger on the Charge Nurses face when we arrived at the hospital, I think it was probably longer than the fingertip was worth.

One more thing about pain; if you need to take pain medication before you go to the hospital to help control your pain, take it. Do not make yourself suffer so the nurse can see you in true pain. Tell the triage person that you took medication to control the pain, how much you took, and how long ago.

The same holds true for a fever. Not taking Tylenol for a fever so the nurse can actually see it on her thermometer is just masochistic. Sadistic if you do that with your child. It really helps to write down the time you took the temperature, the reading on the thermometer, the dose of medication you took for it, and the time you took the medication. One of my pet peeves when I worked the emergency room was well meaning parents who let their children stay in pain or maintain a high fever so that I could 'see it for myself'.

If the Emergency Department is very busy and you are not very sick you may be asked to return to the lobby at this point. If so, you will be re-triaged later. There are time frames set out by policy that dictate how often you have to be re-triaged if you are returned to the lobby. You won't be forgotten. The second triage will include the rest of the initial medical exam which includes your medical history (yes they want to know about your tonsillectomy at age 8 now, but not all the gory details about what you spit up afterward or how you could only eat Jell-O for a week when they promised you ice cream).

If you take medications at home on a regular basis, write down the name of the drugs, the amount of drug in the pills(usually mg or unit on the label), the number of pills you are supposed to take, how often you are supposed to take them, and what you take them for. This information should be on the label of the drug bottle.   Write down all of this information, keep it in your wallet or purse along with your Doctors name and phone number. Even if you only take two pills a day and think you can remember them, write them down. When you are sick or stressed you forget things. Having a good list of medications can help the staff figure out what is wrong with you and make sure you get prescribed medication if you are admitted to the hospital. Also, on this list, include any and all drug and food allergies you have. You will be asked for both. Food allergies are not only for the kitchen staff. Food allergies can help determine allergies to some test dyes and drugs that are used in the hospital.

If you are allergic to a medication you will also be asked what type of reaction you had when you took the medication.   Some of the symptoms that the general public consider 'allergic reactions' do not mean you are allergic to that specific drug. Having nausea after taking Erythromycin on an empty stomach is expected as is dizziness after being given Morphine, so your definition of allergic reaction may not be the same as the medical professionals. That is why they ask the question. They will still write down what you tell them but may classify your symptoms post medication ingestion as an 'adverse reaction' instead of as an allergic reaction.

The federal government mandates some of the questions that you will be asked in triage. If you have not been allowed to have your patient support person with you in triage, these two questions are probably the reason. These include questions about whether or not you are abused at home and if you currently feel like killing yourself. While those questions sound a little out there they serve a purpose. There are people who need outside help in their lives that will not seek that help unless it is offered to them first. These questions sound a little out of place when you go to the ED for a stomach-ache but they have saved lives. If you are abused at home and you would like help with that situation, tell the staff honestly when they ask. They will help you find referrals to safe places to live, get you the protection you need, or give you phone numbers for future reference if you are not ready to seek help now. If you are suicidal, tell them. They are there to help you find the counseling you need. Hopefully, you will be able to answer no to both of these questions.

The questioning will include specific questions about what ails you so be prepared to answer those questions. If you have been throwing up they will want to know what you have thrown up. Was it just lunch or was it blood. Maybe it was just icky green or yellow stuff. Did it look like coffee grounds? Did you have diarrhea too? Are you coughing? Is anything coming up when you cough? What color is it? All this helps with the triage as it gives clues as to what is really wrong with you.

An important hint here. Do NOT go to the bathroom to urinate without asking the nurse if they may want a sample. This is one of the most easily avoided delays in emergency room treatment. People are sick, dehydrated, and they can only urinate once every 3 or 4 hours. If you go to the bathroom in the waiting room bathroom you may not be able to go again for hours. No one wants to wait for that, so before you go….ask. You will probably be given a urine cup and told to return it to the counter or save it for the triage nurse. Yes, they will give you a bag to hide it in.

Additionally, if you are having abdominal pain do not eat or drink anything until after you have seen the Doctor. There are multiple reasons for this. Most importantly, some of the things that can cause abdominal pain require surgery. You do not want to have to put a surgery on hold because you ate a candy bar while waiting to see a Doctor for stomach pain. And if you add food or liquid to a stomach that is already upset it is just going to make things worse. The best thing you can do for a stomach that throws up every time you eat something is to NOT EAT anything for a while. It is common sense that you don't want to add a work load to a system that is already having trouble functioning.

So, now you have waited in the lobby with all the screaming children until the chair has left permanent marks on your buttocks and your symptoms have resolved somewhat. You have to go to work tomorrow so you have waited to see the Doctor through all of this. The

Nurse comes into the lobby and calls your name. Do not take your hot chocolate with you into the back. The Nurse, or tech, will take you to a room with a gurney in it and ask you to change into a hospital gown. Arguing that only your ankle hurts from a car accident 3 days ago will not help. The nurse may still demand that you change into a gown. Remember the Doctor or provider who sees you does not know you and, if they are thorough, will want to check the rest of your body for additional injury. I know it looks stupid but put on the gown and ask for a blanket if you are cold. Some ED Doctors will refuse to see patients unless they can examine the patient fully.

Now, make yourself at home. Your waiting time is not expired. You just have a new place, one closer to the action to do it in and with hope of being seen soon. Hopefully, you brought a book from home, a magazine from the lobby, or there is a TV in the room. Entertaining yourself with your cell phone is OK but turn it off AS SOON AS any staff comes into the room. These people are very busy and if you put that phone ahead of seeing them in importance they may just let you finish a whole series of phone calls before they return to the room. They do not have time to teach you cell phone etiquette, so if you wish to get home in this life-time, put the phone down as soon as a caregiver comes into the room. Some hospitals will demand that you turn your phone off before being allowed in the ED. This is the sad result of many years of poor phone etiquette on the part of patients.

What comes next depends on what you told the triage nurse when you came in. All Emergency departments have Protocols that they work under. For instance, if you told the nurse that you have chest pain the staff will do an EKG, start an IV, attach wires to electrodes on your chest, and draw blood, probably before the Doctor sees you. If you told the nurse you are having back or pelvic pain, pee a lot, and have a fever she will want a urine sample before the Doctor sees you. (Aren't you glad you didn't go in the lobby waiting room bathroom 10 minutes ago?)   If you have been throwing up for 4 days and have severe abdominal pain the nurses will start an IV to rehydrate you, draw blood for labs, ask for a urine sample (see I told you) and (maybe) order an x-ray.   All of this is done because certain illnesses present with similar symptoms and they are trying to save you, and the Doctor, some time. The idea is that it will be easier for the Doctor to tell you what is wrong with you if he has all those test results in hand before he sees you. If the Nurses start an IV before the Doctor sees you they either think you need fluid (think dehydration. Were you throwing up?) or that you may need medication soon (Are you in excruciating pain?). Some of the more serious illnesses have more extensive Protocols. If you are concerned about what the staff is doing or why, ask. The staff will be more than happy to explain to the why to you. Remember from the earlier chapter that the knowledge of what is being done to you is one of the Patient Rights guaranteed by law.

All the tests are done, the results are back, and the IV is running in. Finally, the Doctor or medical practitioner comes in. A really good Emergency Physician will not only take the time to ask you what seems like a thousand questions but will explain to you at this time what he thinks may be wrong with you and what the hospital staff is going to do about it. If he doesn't for some reason, ask. Once again, you have a right to know everything that the hospital is finding out and what they are doing for you. After the Doctor discusses all of this with you, he will leave. Hopefully, he or she has already figured out what is wrong with you and is writing your discharge instructions and a prescription to be sent home which will make you feel better soon. Even if this is the case you will have to wait for a little while longer while the nurses complete the paperwork. A Nurse will then come into your room with discharge paperwork which tells you your medical problem, educational materials which explain your condition in whatever your primary language is, possibly a prescription to make you feel better, a list of medications that you normally take and any new ones that have been added to your regime. You have the right to ask for copies of your labs and other tests they have run. You, or your Doctor's office, can also request these later but it will be a more time consuming process involving the medical records department and signed releases. Also, if you were given any Opiate pain medications during this process you will not be allowed by staff to drive or walk home by yourself. They do not want to get sued. You will be required to produce a driver to take you home. If you have your advocate with you, this should present no problem.

If you are sick enough to stay in the hospital, and statistics show that 40% of all ED patients are admitted to the hospital, the Doctor will have the nurses call the House Supervisor for a bed assignment for you in the appropriate unit while he calls the admitting physician to make sure there is a Doctor to care for you while you are 'in house'. This will, again, result in you waiting. Nothing in a hospital happens fast. There are simply too many variables in hospitals to make things happen fast. First, the Supervisor has to make sure she has a bed to put you in and that it is clean and appropriate to what is wrong with you. Second, she will need to make sure she has a nurse to take care of you and that your nurse, or her floor supervisor, has the time to do an admission assessment and all of the paperwork that goes along with it. When this has been accomplished the House Supervisor will arrange for someone to take you from the Emergency Department to your newly assigned room. There used to be a huge delay with the exchange and review of paperwork but now that all of the paperwork is computerized this shouldn't be a problem. But do not be surprised if you have to wait for a bed to become available. Hospitals are cutting costs which means no spare staff to take in new patients at a moment's notice. Emergency room holds have become so common that there are even specific computer codes for this phenomena. You may have to wait until someone gets well and gets out before you get an available bed.

If you need to go to another hospital for specialized care the Doctor will talk to a Doctor that practices at that facility and the nurses will call the house Supervisor at that hospital for a bed assignment and arrange for an ambulance to take you there. They will not let you drive there by private car unless you sign a form that says you refused medical care and advice. No one wants the liability of a patient dying while driving to another hospital for specialized care. Take the ambulance.

Your insurance should pay for most of it and if you are sick it is easier to sleep on a gurney in an ambulance than sit in a car. Any transfer between hospitals takes time. Try to be patient. (Pun intended!)

"But I wanted the quiet room with a view…." Or admission to a Med/Surg floor

The Medical/Surgical floor is the part of the hospital where the majority of patients are admitted. It is designed for patients that are too sick to go home but not sick enough to go to one of the specialty floors. However, depending on the size of the hospital you can also end up on a specialized medical or surgical floor. There are so many names and variations of areas for this level of care that I could not name all of them. A lot of it depends on the types of Doctors that admit patients to that specific hospital. For instance, I once worked in a hospital that served an elderly population and because of that had 4 Orthopedic Surgeons who operated there. The hospital had an entire floor dedicated to patients recovering from Orthopedic surgery; lots of broken hips. Because of the large percentage of specific types of patients the nurses were highly skilled in the proper application of post-operative devices for healing bones. Administration of pain medications were given at levels that still allowed the physical therapist to work with the patients during the day, and the hospital maintained a higher percentage of nurses aids to help patients that were elderly and had mobility problems. It was a very efficient place to receive care if you had a broken bone. The same hospital, however, only had a 4 bed Obstetric ward because there were not that many babies being born in the elderly community. Hospitals are all different in this regard.

Most medical/surgical floors are general care and treat patients of all types. Their primary function is to get you well enough to go home. The TV version of the hospital where Dr. Welby admitted patients to a hospital for 'a little rest' is a total fantasy, especially in this modern age. Insurance companies are not going to pay for "rest" and hospitals are businesses. Rooms are crowded with equipment and, even if you are lucky enough to score that quiet, private room, hospitals are noisy, 24-hour working businesses.

Your room will contain a bed, lights over the bed, brighter 'exam' lights so the Doctor can actually see that rash you are complaining of, a rolling table that can straddle the bed, a nightstand, plus medical hookups in the wall. Medical hookups are things like Oxygen outlets, suction canisters (these are like a little vacuum for sucking up icky things like vomit), and electrical outlets painted red that go to a generator (In case the electricity goes out). If you are on a floor where they want to watch your heart beat there will probably be different monitors over the bed that serve that purpose although sometimes there is just a little electrical transmitter, about the size of a really fat cell phone, that sits in that weird little pocket on the front of your hospital gown. (You always wondered what that was for, didn't you?)

There will probably be a chair in the room and a bathroom, although some hospitals will make you share your bathroom with connecting rooms or other beds in your room. Yes, there is a good possibility that you will have at least one other bed and person in your room with you. This practice is being phased out in the more modern hospitals due to privacy issues and hospital acquired infections spreading from patient to patient. There will also be a TV hanging up there on the wall for you to watch and a giant remote control which makes not only the TV work but also will adjust the position of your bed and turn on the nurse call light. Don't expect fancy cable TVs or surround sound. The speakers are usually located in the side rails of the bed or on the giant control/nurse call light thing so that you can hear it without bothering the guy in the bed next to you. And, turn off the TV when the Doctor comes into the room. It is very difficult to talk to a patient about their prognosis when they are watching America's funniest bloopers over your shoulder. Most Doctors keep the TV watching phenomena in the same category as cell phone chats and won't react well to this rudeness.

The bed you will be in will be much more comfortable than the gurneys in the emergency department and a whole lot less comfortable than the bed you have at home. Hospital beds are designed to hold sick people which means they have a washable cover over the mattress and big rails on either side that can be pulled up to keep you from falling out (or getting out if the nurses think you are confused). The bed can change position using that weird control device that also controls the aforementioned TV or by pushing the little arrows on the side of the bed. Another variable. Some of the newer beds can be adjusted all the way up into a lounge chair position which is about as uncomfortable as it sounds.

One of the newer bed contraptions that hospitals have come up with have air bladders in the mattresses which inflate and deflate at different intervals. The idea behind these is to reduce the incidence of bedsores from people lying in one position for too long. I do not think that the inventor of these mattresses ever tried actually sleeping on one. While they are useful for patients who are unconscious and cannot move themselves around to protect against bedsores they are very loud when you are lying on them. You can hear the pumps blow up the mattress and then you can hear it release in a low hissing sound. The motion of the bed is also very uncomfortable when you are trying to rest. If you get one of these beds you can request a regular mattress or ask that the bed be turned off if it keeps you awake. The staff will have already rated your chances of developing a bedsore on a standardized chart which includes things like your nutritional status and how alert you are. If you request a regular bed and it is denied it could have to do with your 'score' on these charts.

Bathrooms in hospital rooms are very utilitarian and easy to clean, which in layman's terms means they are ugly. No custom tile here. If you are lucky enough to have a private shower there will probably be one of those little fold down seats in there which help when you don't feel well. There will also be a nurse call light on the wall in case you get to the bathroom and find you are too sick or weak to get back to bed on your own and you didn't bring an advocate. All hospital bathrooms have hand rails for holding onto. Use them. They are there for a reason and if you are in the hospital you are sick or injured. Don't take a chance on falling.

I would be remiss if I didn't address the nurse call light issue. There will be at least two nurse call lights in your room plus a code blue light. Don't confuse them. One brings the nurse or other patient care provider, the other brings a very excited code team with a code cart. The code team won't be happy if you called them by accident. Pushing the regular call light does not mean someone is going to come running into the room. Hospital staff does not just sit out at the desk and wait for the lights to call them in. They all have other patients that they are caring for. The nurse or aid will get into the room or answer you on a speaker as soon as they can. That little light turns on a very annoying alarm and little flashing light at the nurse's station, which will keep reminding them you need them. If the indicator light on your end of the device goes out and no one comes into your room within 5 minutes, push it again. In hospitals, as elsewhere, the squeaky wheel gets the oil. Unless you have become one of those demanding patients that hits the call light to have the nurse change channels on the TV for you, she or he will be in as soon as they can be.

Usually there is a white write-on board of some type hanging on the wall in hospital rooms. This is for writing the day of the week, your nurse's name, Doctors name, and other little tidbits of information that you probably won't remember unless it is written up there. It sounds silly to a healthy person but three days in a hospital and Tuesday very easily seems like Saturday.

There will also be a telephone in your room. These are placed there for local calls and probably will not work should you decide to catch up with Aunt Bertha in Australia. If you have a legitimate need to make a long distance call and either don't have a cell phone or it doesn't work in the room, call the operator and tell her. Hospitals are able to connect you to a line which has long distance capability. Don't abuse this. I have seen hospitals add phone charges to bills for patients who used their time in the hospital to call everyone they know.

Your cell phone, by the way, may not work in the hospital. The electronics on different floors can interfere with your phone signal. Also, I should mention, the reason that most hospitals have it posted that you may not use your cell phone is not because it interferes with their electronics, although that is the excuse most often given and it was at one time a fact. I cannot say this enough: Cell phone use is discouraged in hospitals because of simple phone courtesy. There are some patients who will not stop a conversation with Joe Blow about the game next weekend when the Doctor or the nurse comes into the room. I know that you think your phone call is hugely important but you can call your friend back. Doctors and Nurses are very busy during the course of the day. They do not have time, or the patience for that matter, to stand and wait with your pills or lab work for you and Joe to finish your game theory conversation. Do not expect them too. I have seen Doctors put patients to the end of the day list because they didn't have the common courtesy to terminate their conversation when the Doctor wanted to talk to them. Nurses too. They have a busy day and can't stand by with your pills while you chat with Grandma. And, yes, they do have to watch you take those pills.

Speaking of nurses, that cute little bouncy nurse that you see on TV who flashes cleavage while she lovingly gives bed bathes and helps patients fluff their pillows is a myth. I am not sure where that idea of nursing care came from. Nurses work hard; have always worked hard and have little time for fluffing of pillows. (Pillow fluffing is one of those reasons that you brought your advocate with you.)

By the way, I in no way wish to offend anyone for my use of the word 'she' for the nurse or 'he' for the Doctor.   There is a large increase in the number of men that are choosing nursing as a viable career opportunity. Job security is pretty much guaranteed (there will always be sick people) and the pay has increased to a point in most areas of the country where you can actually support a family in good style with it. This was traditionally a female career position and most nurses are still of the female persuasion so, at the risk of offending some of the incredibly talented male nurses I know, I will use that descriptive for nurses since our language does not contain pronouns that include both sexes.

All hospitals differ in the number of patients that are assigned to each nurse unless it is regulated by state law, as in the case of California. Even then, if you have caring supervisors, there may be some variance to staffing numbers based on the "acuity" of the patients. (Acuity is a fancy way of determining how much time the nurse should have to spend caring for the patient. I know, it sounds cold, but remember this is a business.)

Most General medical floors will assign 4 to 5 patients to every nurse. That is a busy work day especially if the nurses at that hospital do 'primary care', which means there are no Certified Nursing Assistants to help with patient needs. To help you understand this a little more let's take a look at what the average nurse does in a day for her patients, remembering that in most hospitals the shifts are 8 to 12 hours long.

An average day for a General Care Nurse starts with taking report from the off going nurse or nurses that cared for her patients the night before. This process usually takes around 30 minutes. Then she will make notes on all of these patients to help her organize her workday. Next, that nurse will need to go through the patients charts and verify all of the medications each patient is scheduled to receive during her shift by reading through the Doctors progress notes and order sheets. She will also look at the labs that were drawn at some ungodly hour of the morning to see if there are any abnormal numbers that need to be called to the physicians notice. All of this needs to be done by 9:00 which is when most patients are scheduled to receive their morning medications. If there is no CNA the nurse will also have to find time in there somewhere to make sure that all of her patients received their breakfast and that it is the correct type of diet advised for that patient. (Tired yet?)

Most nurses make little handwritten charts for themselves to keep track of which patients get which medications at what time. There are innumerable ways to verify medications be given to the correct patient, most require some documentation. In addition to that, it is the nurse's job to make sure that they are given on time. Being that this is a hospital which holds sick people almost all patients have medications that need to be given. The nurse has to get the individual medications from the medication room or cart, take them into the patient's room, verify that it is the right patient in the right bed, and stay there until the medications are taken or given. One of the new ways of doing this is by use of what appears to be a grocery store scanner with which the nurse will scan first a your wrist band and then the medication. It is a safety precaution and against the rules for a nurse to take two patients medications from the medication cart at the same time. If there has been an error with the patient's medications she has to contact the in-house pharmacist to see that it is corrected and then document it in a special form. Some high-risk medications have to be signed off by two nurses before they are given which means waiting for another nurse, who is trying to accomplish this same task with her patients, to have the time to come into the room, check the medication, check the orders for the patient, and sign.

IV medications take extra time with new tubing every few days and medication pumps which need programing. The IV itself has to be restarted every few days to reduce the risk of infection of the area where the needle goes under the skin. Blood transfusions take even longer with a two nurse double checking requirement and specialized tubing, required IV catheter sizes, and loads of paperwork to make sure the right blood is given to the right patient. Should the patient request medication that is not on the chart, even something simple like aspirin or Tylenol, the nurse will have to track down the Doctor to get the order added to the chart.

After the medications are given there are bed baths waiting to happen, bed linens that need to be changed, call lights that need answering, Doctors making rounds that want the nurses attention, and lunches to be delivered. In addition to all of this the nurse may have to take patients down to other floors for x-rays, CT scans, MRI's. Plus, she is responsible for discharging patients that are well enough to go home or need to go to another facility. If the nurse is lucky she will have a social worker on hand to arrange for at home equipment and transportation but she is still responsible for making sure all of that is ready before the patient leaves the hospital. Then she is responsible for admitting patients to fill the beds left empty by those discharges. The paper work involved in both of those processes is incredibly long and involved. Now, add in the time involved in talking to patients and families, answering call lights, talking to Doctors, answering calls from the pharmacy or lab, changing wound dressings, restarting IV catheters, lines, and bags, helping patients up to the bathroom so they don't fall, and reporting off to other staff. There is an old joke in nursing about nurses wearing bladder catheters and bags attached to their legs because they don't have time to go to the bathroom. There are days where that seems a viable option. Hopefully there is a good charge nurse on the floor so the nurse had a few minutes to eat lunch or a snack to keep energy levels up.

*Care Provider Point- Now that I have hopefully helped people understand what a nurse does all day long I would like to address the medical staff. Doctors, Nurses, Aids, Techs and anyone else that comes in contact with a patient in the hospital. There are a few consistent complaints that I heard from patients over the years in reference to the staff in hospitals. The most common complaint that I get from patients has to do with communication. They felt that staff was either talking too fast, were incomprehensible, or, more commonly, treating them like they left their brains at home. After becoming a patient and a patient advocate myself I realize the complexity of this issue. I am a Registered Nurse trained in Emergency and Critical Care who works as a Hospital Supervisor and my husband is a retired Emergency Room physician; yet the times we did not identify ourselves as such we were treated like, quite honestly, idiots. Staff, don't treat your patients this way. It's insulting. Yes, they are sick but they are not stupid. When you are explaining things to your patients tell them to stop you if they don't understand and then be truthful and fluid in your speech. If you don't know the answer to a question you are asked tell them so and then go find the answer. Don't lie to people thinking they are not going to know the difference. You do not know who that person in the bed is in their life outside the hospital. You could be talking to Scientist, a Judge, or a Doctor. As House Supervisor when I was called into a patients room to explain something that my staff should have already explained two or three times I always asked the person in the bed and their advocate what they do for a living. It really helps to adjust the level of communication and explanation of medical procedure. It also saves time since if you explain it truthfully and on the patients level the first time you won't have to repeat yourself later. Or the Supervisor will not have to spend his or her time re-explaining something that you should have told the patient in the first place. This goes for physicians too. We know you are busy but these people are entrusting you with their lives. That type of trust should make you feel humble and it deserves the time to make sure the communication is clear.

I have to digress here for one of my favorite 'lack of communication stories' as it so perfectly exemplifies the lack of priority given to communication with patients. At the time I was working in a hospital in a closed community in the mid-west after spending years in California where I was exposed to a phenomenal number of cultures and the practices that go with the varied life styles. During early morning report I was told that one of the patients I was being assigned to was a 'little slow' and that his family was also 'not quite with it'. The patient's last name indicated possible Hispanic heritage so I asked if an interpreter had been called in. The off going nurse assured me, rather indignantly, that they had used the language interpretation phone and that the Doctor spoke some Spanish. She said they 'just didn't get it'. When I walked into the room to introduce myself to the family I was amazed to see an entire Hmong family sitting before me, some in traditional garb. Excuses to be made for the staff would be that there simply was no Hmong or any other of the Southeast Asian immigrants in that part of the country yet and they had never been exposed to that culture but the truth was that the staff was careless in their communication. I took one look at the family and asked them one simple word, "Hmong?" Their faces lit up and the matriarch jumped up and grabbed my hand. She was so thankful that finally someone got it. I returned with the interpreter phone and the Doctor. Things were explained in their own language and dialect. Hmong are a very polite, respectful people and this wonderful family had simply sat there nodding their heads in agreeable fashion while all of these kind strangers kept talking to them in languages they did not understand. What a simple fix and a wonderful lesson! Take the time to talk to your patients.

Another complaint that I frequently received was from elderly people who were hard of hearing and had been assigned caregivers with heavy accents. That is never a good combination. We would end up with very angry elderly people who could not understand a word the Doctor or Nurse was saying. Communication is a complicated skill at best and it takes time and caring. Personnel in charge of assignments of staff to patients should take factors like this into account. So many problems could be avoided by taking a little time to insure that communication is arranged for optimal ease of the patients.

I spent several paragraphs explaining to the person in the bed what the caregivers were doing with their time. Now let's take a paragraph to examine what the patient's day is like. First of all, they probably got very little restful sleep the night before. Hospitals are noisy places at all hours of the day and night. Night nurses very rarely are sensitive to the sleep patterns of their patients. Waking up a non-critical patient to take a blood pressure and ask them how they feel at 2:00 in the morning is just cruel. If you have to have that BP try to be as nonintrusive as possible. You don't need all the lights on to check a blood pressure and the patient does not want to chit chat with you about how your night is going. The person in the bed is sick and tired. They want to sleep. Close the door on your way out! Unless your patient is a fall risk or too confused to push the call light. A little privacy please!

Breakfast usually arrives to the floors around 7:30. Nurses I know this is a busy time for you but have you ever tried to eat cold oatmeal when you don't feel good anyway? If you don't have a CNA, deliver the trays yourself. Take the time to introduce yourself. An early morning helping of friendly face and warm food will go a long way towards making your patients happier. And happy patients are really much easier to care for.

To a patient that is not very ill but not well enough to go home, days in the hospital can seem like forever. Stop and think about it. You are too weak to get out of bed, the TV is boring, you have read three novels and now you have a headache.   You can't sleep because the nurse left the door open and the noise is horrific. Breakfast was far from inviting but the vanilla pudding that came with the dried out sandwich they served for lunch suddenly seems very exciting. You are forced to lie in an uncomfortable bed all day long waiting for the Doctor to come in and decide if you can go home. No one knows when the Doctor will be in. You've ask four different people who were all dressed alike but they all told you that they were not your nurse. Medical care in hospitals would improve immensely if the caregivers just took the time to imagine what it is like to be a patient in that bed. How would you want to be treated?

I'm really not sure where the practice of blood draws at 5:00 in the morning came from. Sure, some labs need to be drawn before the patient eats anything and the Doctors like to have the results of the morning labs before they make rounds but now in the days of the hospitalist it seems a very unnecessary irritant for the patient. Hospitals are there to serve patients, not Doctors. We need to be working around what is good for the person in the bed not the person who is healthy enough to be taking care of them.

Back to the Patient: One more important point here. Nosocomial is the name given to infections that are acquired by patients while they are in the hospital.   This is a huge problem yet few patients have ever been advised of the risks. Did your caregiver wash her hands or use the antibacterial rub mounted on the wall when they came into your room? If not you need to ask them to do so and not be shy about it. Thousands of people die every year from infections that they 'caught' while they were in the hospital. Thousands more are treated for infections that are very difficult to eradicate. Hospitals are germy places and some of the germs that breed there are very scary little bugs. MRSA (Methicillin Resistant Staphylococcus aureus) is just one of these scary germs. Staph aureus has lived on people since before we knew what bacteria were but, due to the overuse of antibiotics in our culture, they have mutated into deadly strains. The news media has grabbed this and refers to it as a flesh eating bacteria. Every year more and more of these frightening strains of bacteria are being found as they continue to mutate with the over use of antibiotics.

If you are in a hospital that is cautious about preventing nosocomial infections you were probably given a nasal swab on admission (a test similar to the nasal swab test for the flu). If you are found to be positive you will be placed in 'Isolation', which is a private room and requires anyone coming into your room to wear a gown, gloves and sometimes a mask as a precaution to spreading the infection to other patients and staff. Do not take this lightly! If you a placed in a room with someone who is coughing, sneezing, or has open oozing sores, ask to be moved to another room. Hospitals are usually very diligent about these hospital acquired infections and take precautions but this is serious enough that you should remain vigilant. If you are in the hospital you already have a suppressed immune system and are therefore, susceptible to additional infections.

Also, on the same subject, you have the right to refuse anything that the hospital wishes to do to you. It is your body. For instance, if the nurse comes in with a Foley catheter (a device which drains urine from the bladder to a bag on the side of the bed) ask the necessity for it. These are used to measure the amount of urine people put out every day which can be instrumental in determining diagnosis but they are also inserted in patients which may not have a huge medical need for them. If you can walk to the toilet, the nurse can measure your urine output from one of those little white 'hats' that sit in the toilet. For men it is even easier in the form of a urinal which is a little plastic bottle designed for a man to urinate into. Granted it is much more convenient for the nurse to only have to empty that bag once a shift then to come into your room every two hours to help you up to the commode or pick up the urinal you dropped but anything that is inserted into your body creates a possible pathway for bacteria to enter the body. The same is true for IV's. Your skin is your first defense against infection   A nurse who is not good at establishing IV's will leave an opening for bacteria to enter into your body every time she pokes you with another needle.

We have a friend who was transferred from one hospital to a second for legitimate medical reasons. He needed an IV and the first hospital had established one. A nurse in the second hospital did not like the type of Angio-Cath (a type of needle) that the first hospital had used and removed it. Our friend was dehydrated which means his veins were deflated, not enough blood flowing through there to plump up for an IV to be inserted. They poked him 5 times before an Anesthesiologist was called in to restart what was a viable IV. In addition to the pain and discomfort of the needle sticks it also left him with 5 extra openings for bacteria to get under his skin. He should have refused to let her pull the IV. Most hospitals have rules about restarting IV's every 3 to 4 days anyway to prevent IV tubing from causing an infection. Our friend now had 5 less areas available for the necessary IV to be restarted.

I know that it is very difficult to stand up to medical professionals especially when you don't feel well and just want to be taken care of. But, it is your body, the only one you have, that is being poked and prodded by these people. If something does not seem right, ask. If you don't like the answer, ask a supervisor or the Doctor. It is primarily your responsibility and definitely in your best interest for you to take care of your body since you live in it.

The Intensive Care Unit or ICU

There are good things and bad things about ending up in ICU. The worst of these, of course, is that you are sick enough to end up in ICU. ICU is reserved for patients who need critical care. Vital signs are monitored frequently if not constantly, sometimes through intrusive devices (yes, there really are such things as rectal probes). The people in ICUs frequently have a pharmacopeia of drugs hanging from poles that surround the beds. It can be a very frightening place to be. So let's examine first the good points.

First of all, in the ICU you will most likely have a private room and while the walls will be made of glass the nurses will close these doors behind them when the leave the room. Depending on your condition they can even be talked into pulling the curtains to give you more privacy. You will have a private toilet, although no shower, right in the room and not far from the bed. The nursing ratios are very different for ICU and you will probably only have to share your nurse with only one other patient. That means they will be able to focus more of their time on you. Unfortunately, it also means that you are sick enough to require that extra care. Also, Doctors usually start rounds in the ICU which means you have to wait less time to see them. Unfortunately, by the time you are well enough to appreciate all of this you will probably be moved to another floor.

ICU's are very busy places. They are highly specialized and very organized. The nurses that choose to work in ICU's have very specialized training in drugs, equipment, and diseases. They have chosen to seek out this specialized training in order to work with the sickest of the sick. Staff wise, in the ICU, you are in very good hands.

All nurses are attracted to specific areas of care that align with their own personality types. I used to illustrate this by telling the story of how in one of the hospitals I worked in the various departments decorated for Christmas. In the ED, the nurses created their own designs on multi colored balls which were hung at varying lengths, helter-skelter from the ceiling of the department. Med/Surg nurses had multi-colored balls but they were clustered on the counter and hanging on a tree. ICU nurses had gold and silver balls that were hung from the ceiling on carefully measured lengths of ribbon (also silver and gold) in exacting positions which created a flowing (yet very straight) design. It was an interesting phenomena.

ICU is one area of the hospital where you will not be allowed to have your advocate with you except within limited windows. If you are in the ICU you are very sick or need lots of care. Life and death are always a fine balance in the ICU. If you are able to communicate make sure that you tell staff that when the Doctor makes rounds you want to have your advocate with you. On the advocate's part, this takes lots of commitment since they will be spending hours in the waiting room doing just that; waiting and waiting. While I find it discomforting that if you are in the ICU you are probably in a condition where you require an advocate

102

I am comforted because I understand the level of training that these nurses have and the depths of their commitment to their patients. Hopefully, before you ever get admitted to an ICU you have your Medical Power of Attorney drawn up. This will empower whomever you have chosen to speak for you and the nurses will keep that person informed of your progress.

Another issue I will address here is your living will which your lawyer should have encouraged you to draw up while he was doing your Power Of Attorney. This is a document that will tell medical personnel, family, your advocate, and whoever holds your power of attorney how much you want your body to endure should you die. For example, do you want people to do CPR on you? CPR can save lives but it is a very traumatic procedure. Your baseline medical condition should be closely considered before filling one of these out. This is never an easy subject so you probably have not spoken to anyone about it. I strongly suggest that you take one to your physician and have him explain what procedures are appropriate. Lawyers are not medically trained and I have seen some living wills that make no medical sense and even contradict themselves. People's wishes sometimes are ignored if they don't make sense since legally Doctors are required to try to save you unless you have paperwork stating otherwise.

You should also be aware of what CPR and resuscitation efforts entail. This is not like on TV where they zap you once, pump on your chest for 2 minutes, and you get up and walk home. CPR is the act of breathing for someone and squeezing their heart after they have died in an effort to bring them back. It does sometimes work but it also causes trauma to the chest cavity. The C in CPR stands for Cardiac and the act of pumping the heart involves someone pushing on the chest wall to a depth of 2-3 inches. Most often bones are broken in the process. P stands for Pulmonary or lungs. This portion involves someone forcing air down into the lungs. Eventually a tube is inserted in the airway to protect it. This is called Intubation. The process also sometimes involves the utilization of electricity in some deadly rhythms to stop the heart and allow it to reset itself (hopefully). The electricity can also cause burns. There are IV's involved and a plethora of very strong drugs. Yes, the process can restart a heart that has stopped and save a life but the reality of the process is brutal and needs to be considered before signing the paperwork that tells people what you do and don't want done. This paperwork also tells people when to stop trying to save you which is really important. The brain can only live for 5 minutes without blood flow. Restarting a heart when it has been stopped for too long can mean being kept alive by machines because the brain is in a vegetative state. Talk to your Doctor. Get his or her opinion, based on your medical condition, what measures would be appropriate for you.

Now that I have frightened you I will also tell you that sometimes doctors admit people to ICU when they need labor intensive treatments, as they are familiar with the heavy load of the floor nurses. Once again the staffing in ICU is usually one Nurse for every two patients which means these nurse have more time to spend with patients. If you are admitted to ICU you have the right to ask why this department was chosen for you.

When you get better you will be moved to another floor, usually a step down unit, which means you don't need ICU anymore but are not ready for the Med/Surg floor unless it is a very small hospital. These step down units are usually Telemetry floors where you have to wear that heart monitor in the little pocket and have your vital signs taken every 4 hours. Assignments for nurses on step down units are usually 3 to 4 patients to a nurse. Frighteningly, the less you see your nurse the better you probably are. How long you stay on this floor will depend on your progress and on your Doctors opinion of your medical condition. You may soon be lucky enough to go home to your own bed.

The Laboratory

The laboratory in the hospital is one of those places that most people never see in its entirety. When your blood is ordered as an out-patient you go in the front section and sit on the hard chair with the arm holder while your blood is drawn. This is the face of the lab and does not even hint at the extensive machinery and exhausting equipment that lurks in the back.

The Lab is where all of those substances and other things that come out of or are removed from your body are taken. When that perky little phlebotomist wakes you up at two in the morning to draw your blood, this is where she and her cart originated from and where she will return to after she draws your blood. When the nurse has you relieve yourself in one of those funny looking little plastic things that fit inside the toilet; this is where she will send whatever comes out of you. If the surgeon cuts something out of you, this is where it ends up.

This is the area where there are people who will look at it under the microscope and run it through machines. Depending on what "it" is they may freeze it and slice it, or send it to other labs. The oven (incubator) that keeps the icky stuff that came out of your wound warm are kept here to help grow more of what even caused your infection in the first place.

This is also the place where they check your blood sample to figure out your blood type. The replacement blood, if ordered, has to come through here and be checked before it can find its way into your veins. Blood, Platelets, and plasma are double checked here and labeled with multiple identifiers before nurses are called to pick it up. The lab will require that the nurse have your name, birthdate, record number and blood type before the allowing her to sign for the blood and take it back to the floor.

The lab is staffed with clerks, phlebotomists, laboratory technicians, and Doctors of Clinical Pathology who oversee the smooth functioning of this complicated place.

The "stuff" that comes out of you is sent here in biohazard containers and bags marked with your name and other information. The orders for the information that the Doctor would like to obtain from this "stuff" is sent with it or is already in the lab computer waiting. It will be processed by the members of this team and the information will be sent back to your nurse and Doctor in the form of a print out or computer sheet that break the information down into what is normal and what is not normal.

You have a right to see this information. It is part of your chart. Do not be concerned if some of the numbers are outside of what the lab calls its "Normal values". Everyone has slight fluctuations in what is normal for their body. The lab will call your nurse, who in turn will call your Doctor, if your lab values are different enough from the normal levels to need immediate concern.

The information contained in the fluctuations of your lab values can help your Doctor with diagnosing any abnormalities that are present in the function of your body. Mind that I said 'help your Doctor". These numbers are not magic medicine. They are part of a giant puzzle that your Doctor will put together with the other pieces of the puzzle in order to help you feel better.

Most lab tests can be done rapidly but most take a minimum of several hours to have results. If the test being run is more complicated, requires special machines, or involves infections it may take up to several days to have even preliminary results.

Cultures are groups of different bacteria that are grown out of substances from your body in incubators in the laboratory. For instance, if you have a bladder infection the lab can detect the presence of certain cells in your urine with a simple dip strip test. But, the test required to determine if the bacteria growing in your bladder will respond to specific antibiotics will take days. If you are being treated for a suspected infection your Doctor will not wait for these lab result to begin treating you. You will be given doses of antibiotics that kill a "wide spectrum" of possible bacteria that could be causing your illness. The medications will be adjusted later if the germs that grow out are resistant to or don't respond to what you are taking.

If you are treated in the Emergency Department and samples are sent to the lab to be 'cultured' you will be called if anything grows out that needs treatment other than the one you were released with. If you are a worrier, you can call the lab for results but they may require you to go into the medical records department to get the results. The HIPPA privacy laws have made hospitals very nervous about releasing this type of information without confirmation that you are the person the "stuff" came out of in the first place.

When your Doctor sends you to the hospital lab as an outpatient he sends you with an order which tells the lab to send the results to his or her office. Your Doctor will call you if there are any results that you need to be aware of. You will probably have more luck obtaining information about your medical lab values from your Doctor's office than from the lab.

The people that work in this department are only seen when they are visiting the bedside with a tray of needles and tubes. Like most hospital staff, they really care about their profession. If you have questions about what tests they are doing, ask them. They will not be able to tell you anything about your specific condition but they can tell what tests they are doing on your blood, urine, etc. Also, don't ask them to interpret your results. They do not have access to your chart, information about your condition, or the schooling to interpret those results as regards to your specific condition.

"I can see right through you…" or the Radiology Department

The simple x-rays they used to shoot back in the day to see if you broke your arm when you fell of the swing set are not that simple anymore. They are definitely better regulated and, thus, safer than the x-rays of yesteryear. New technology and machines have evolved that can pick out minute details of things that are deep inside your body.   The simple x-ray machine that used to show just your bony structure has evolved into CT scans, PET scans, MRI's, Ultrasounds, and now DSA. All of these are tests where differing forms of energy are sent through your body. The various densities of the tissues of your body reflect or block these various forms of energy which results in images that Doctors are trained to translate.

If one of these diagnostic tests is ordered for you that is the way it will be announced. What do those letters stand for? CT stands for Computed Tomography, PET is Positron emission tomography, MRI stands for Magnetic resonance imaging, and an Ultrasound is just that; sound waves, and DSA is digital Subtraction Angiography. And what is the difference? I'll give you the short version here which will probably give some Radiologist nightmares.

CT scan, which is in commonly used for diagnosis assistance these days, is a full depth, cross sectional, 3-D image of your innards. It allows a Doctor specifically trained in Radiology to see if everything is where it is supposed to be and that there is nothing extra in there, like air, fluid or cellular mutations.

A PET is a scan which uses a radiographic dye and tracks it through the body to a specific area. It does not show detailed structural imaging but rather "hot spots" of increased metabolic activity such as cancer.

MRI uses Magnetic fields and radio waves to show more specific details of soft tissue. MRI's are commonly used for accessing damage to ligaments and tendons. This is the test they will do if you injure a joint for instance. They are also commonly used to closely inspect questionable tissue that shows up on x-rays.

An ultrasound (or sonogram) uses incredibly high sound waves to determine distances and find objects without destroying or damaging the tissue the way that excessive radiation from other tests can. Examples of use would be for examining a pregnancy and looking more closely at questionable tissue from mammograms.

A DSA is a type of fluoroscopy and is a way of looking at veins and arteries without the interference of other structures. Fluoroscopy is an image that shows movement inside of you. For instance, an angiogram, where the Doctor injects a dye into your veins to watch the blood flow through specific arteries and veins.

There are innumerable other tests out there that are specific to what Doctors are looking for in your body. This is a very specialized area of investigative medicine and I am by no means an expert in it. I do know that the amount of radiation that will enter your body with these different tests varies greatly and should be a consideration on your part prior to the tests especially if they are ordered on a child. If your Doctor orders one of these tests, ask him to explain it to you. Ask what he is looking for and exactly what the test entails. In addition to the radiation you are exposed to some of these tests also include injection of dyes into the blood stream. The technician will ask you about specific allergies, including food allergies, before injecting you with these dyes. Be honest with them. If you have kidney problems you need to make sure that the technician is aware of that fact as these dyes can cause additional damage to the kidneys.

Once again, the technicians that do these tests are professionally trained. They can answer your general questions about the tests being done but cannot interpret the tests for you. You do have a right to see the results of these tests and even have copies of them. Do not expect to be able to see what your Doctor has seen. If you want copies, ask the procedure for obtaining them. It is usually fairly simple to print out extra copies but the hospital will probably require another signed release.

"and the pill that Mother gives you……."Medications and the Pharmacy

As a house supervisor one of my responsibilities was to document any medication errors that came to light during my shifts. I was very proud of the fact that these errors did not seem to occur very frequently and that my staff appeared meticulous in their administration of medications.   As the wife of a patient I was horrified to find that medication errors occurred during every visit that my husband and I made to the hospital. The frustrating part of this was that the medications that were most frequently messed up were not the medications that were new to the patient and ordered by the Doctor that was treating the patient in house but rather home medications that should be continued during a hospital stay.

To understand this a little better we need to look at the process in having home medications transferred into the world of the hospital.

The first responsibility, of course, is that of the patient. It is the patients' responsibility to have in their possession a copy of all of their home medications, the dosage they take, the number of times a day they take it, and (hopefully) an understanding of why they take those medications. This includes supplements and herbal remedies. This last part is very important. You should know what you are putting into your body and why. You should know the side effects of all medications that you take and what your doctor hopes to accomplish by giving you this specific pill. This includes herbs and supplements. A Doctor or Pharmacist should look over ALL medications and approve, or at least not disapprove, any over the counter medications or supplements that you have in your regimen before you are allowed to take them in the hospital.

In my years of practicing medicine at the bedside I frequently met the patient who had one of those day pill dispenser with a rainbow of non-descript pills rolling around in them. Asking them what medications they take would result in answers such as "I take the little one in the morning, the big one at lunch and the Blue one before bedtime." It was very frustrating that so many patients had so little knowledge of what they were putting into their bodies or why.

Keep an updated list of your medications in your wallet, purse, or taped to the lid of your handy pill dispenser. This is easy to do and will help make the home medication turmoil less turbulent. Providing the nurse with the name of the pharmacy where you get your medications filled is second best as she or he can call the pharmacy to find out what medications you have had filled and how often.

Your next responsibility as a patient is to make sure that the triage nurse or admitting nurse has your complete and accurate list of medications. You cannot watch her add them to your chart to verify they are correctly charted but providing the correct list will help. You also need to make sure that the nurse knows what time of day your take your medications and when the last time that you took them. Some medications work by building up a certain level of the medication in your blood and it is very important to take them as scheduled.

This next part I cannot emphasize enough. If it was possible to print this is huge red letters I would. EVERY time someone brings you a pill or a syringe when you are in the hospital you need to ask what it is and what it is for. Do not take medications without knowing what they are for. It is frighteningly easy for those computer lists of medications to get jumbled or passed over by over worked Doctors who don't know your case. If it doesn't sound right, don't take it! You are still in control of your body and what gets put into it. Your advocate should have a list of medications that you take at home and if you are unable to question the nurse, should be empowered enough to do so on your behalf. It is OK to say 'No' to a new pill until someone explains to you what it is for. This is especially important if you have chronic health issues that are kept in balance by home medications.

If someone tells you that a specific medication is an 'auto-sub' for something you take at home you have the right to obtain medication information before taking it. Not all 'auto-subs' have exactly the same effects as the drugs they are meant to cover for. If you have grave doubts, pick up the bedside phone and call your home pharmacist or private physician.

If you refuse a medication you will have to continue to question it every time the nurse brings you additional pills. Most medications are automatically renewed by the computer on a daily basis.

There are, of course, routes for medications to be delivered to your body other than pills. When you were first admitted to the hospital someone probably stuck a needle in a vein in your arm and either hung a bag of fluid over you that is running into that vein or capped it off with a little extension tail that is taped to your arm. Most people in this modern world run a little on the dehydrated side so an IV is not going to hurt you unless you are for some reason on fluid restrictions. Do you have Congestive Heart failure (commonly called CHF)? Are you in renal failure? If either of those things is true you need to point it out to your nurse so that she can adjust the amount of fluids you are getting accordingly. Bear in mind there are reasons that a Doctor will order you to be given extra fluids even if you have one of those conditions, but once again, if you are concerned; ask.

There are many different types of fluids that are available for IV's. The most common of these is normal saline or NS. The bag probably is just marked with 0.9% on the outside. This is sterile water that has the same amount of sodium (or salt) in it that you normally have in your blood stream. It is used for bolstering the fluid levels that exists inside of your veins. Think of it as topping off your tank in your car. There are other concentrations of fluid that are just saline. There are bags with combinations of saline and dextrose (D5) in them. Hopefully if you have diabetes you have already told your nurse so she does not overload you with sugar. Although, once again, there are reasons for giving diabetics solutions that contain low levels of sugar. There are also solutions that contain combinations of electrolytes (such as potassium).

These can get rather complicated as some are used for pushing fluids into your cells and some are used for pulling fluid off. We would need a whole physiology course here to explain it in detail but you can, of course, ask your nurse why you ae getting what you are getting.

IV or intravenous medications are a whole new challenge. Antibiotics and pain medications are the medications most frequently given through IV access. This is because they work more effectively and the amount you are given is better controlled when they are placed directly into your blood stream. There is also very little delay in the medications taking effect when they bypass your GI track and go directly into the blood stream.

One frequently used form of delivering pain medication to patients in the hospital is medication that is in a pump attached to your IV. You will be given a little button to push when you want to administer your own pain medications (within set parameters) when you need them. The machine will stop giving you medication when you reach the maximum dose ordered by the Doctor. It is a great delivery method which really simplifies the nursing job of providing timely pain medication. If you have maxed out your dose, the machine won't give you anymore drugs, and you feel like you need additional relief you can ask the nurse. She may have additional medications for you on your chart that will fill that need.

Antibiotics that are given through this route are closely monitored. These are very potent drugs. Some of them require blood draws to make sure that the drugs you are being given are building to the needed levels in your bloodstream. Most antibiotics that you are given the first few days you are in the hospital are what they call broad spectrum antibiotics. These kill all kinds of different bacteria. Sometimes these medications are changed when the results of cultures come back from the lab to better combat whatever it is you are fighting.

Most standard medications have an IV form available for use in a hospital. If you are really nauseated or the Doctor does not want anything in your stomach (such as before surgery) you will be given most of your medications this way.

A couple of extra comments on IV's and medications that go into them.   If you have itching in the area of your IV, tell your nurse right away. Especially if she has just recently given you a medication. If you notice redness in the area, again, call your nurse immediately and let her examine the site. If you see blood backing up into the tube, call your nurse. She probably needs to hang a new bag. Swelling at the site of the IV also needs to be addressed.   You should also call your nurse if you see a large air bubble in the IV line. A tiny little bubble will not hurt you but a large amount of air in the IV can kill you.

Don't take chances with your life. You have a right to be the noisy patient. It is your body.

Another route that you can be given medications is an injection or a shot. I know we all hate shots but a well-trained nurse doesn't have to make it hurt. This route for medication takes a shorter time for effect then a pill but is substantially longer then medication given in the IV. Most shots are given in either the upper arm or the buttocks although there are several medications that work better when they are injected into the fat on your stomach. Yes, I know. That sounds horrible but those medications are given through a little tiny needle and not deep. Only into the lining of fat around your middle. (We all knew that had to be good for something!) The process for an injection is pretty simple. Your nurse will wipe the area with alcohol, pinch the surrounding area (this serves two purposes. It seems to make it hurt less and it holds you still.), gently push the needle to the proper depth and then depress the plunger. Pain medications given this way take about 10 to 15 minutes to work.

There is yet another route that nobody likes to think about and that is up your bottom. There are suppositories available for lots of medications.   Medications are absorbed very readily through the lining of your intestinal tract. This is a great way to give medications for nausea as there is no chance of the medication being vomited back up. Yes, it's embarrassing and a little uncomfortable but it works. The suppositories are made of a waxy substance that dissolves with body heat.   They are usually kept in a refrigerator so that they stay solid until the nurse removes them, coats them with slippery stuff, and slides them gently where they will do the most good. If you have body issues, tell you nurse.

Another way you can be given medication is through a little sticky patch that is applied to your skin surface. This is a very slow method of delivering medication but it does work and is used a lot for long term, slow delivery pain medications. Tell your nurse if it itches as some people are allergic to the adhesive in the patch.

Some medications can be inhaled so they are absorbed in the lungs which is a very fast route. These drugs hit your blood stream immediately. That is one of the reason that smokers have such a hard time quitting.

There are, of course, other ways to give medications to a patient but these are the ones you are most likely to encounter. I cannot end this chapter without telling you, yet again, to ask your nurse what the medications are that you are being given. Hospitals are constantly coming up with new ways to make sure that the right drugs get to the right patients but this is still one of the areas where hospitals fall short. If more patients asked what they were being given fewer mistakes would be made.

I need to add some information here on herbs and supplements. Herbs are medications. I repeat; Herbs are medications. Just because your neighbor took an herb for a problem he was having and it made him feel better does not mean that you too should be on that herb. Would you also take his heart pills because he feels better when he takes them?

Herbs do work medically, however, for the most part their action is slower and has a less profound effect on the body than western medicine drugs. Many herbs need to be taken for a long time before their effect is felt. Many modern drugs are simply modified herbs. Herbs were the only medications that were available for centuries. Unfortunately, in the United States western medicine has developed an aversion to treatment by herbs. I do not understand it as for many people herbs work as well as western medicine but with fewer side effects. Some people are more resistant to herbs and, if they were dispensed by an herbalist, would probably require a higher dosage.

The problem with attempting to ignore an entire form of medications has led to an ignorant state where many physicians discount the use of herbs completely. By doing so they are endangering their patients' lives. Herbs not only can have a therapeutic effect but they also can have side effects, cause overdoses, and interact poorly with other medications that the patient is on. It only takes one nurse or Doctor rolling their eyes at a list of medications to make a patient less honest about what they take and what they take it for.

If you are one of the millions of Americans that take an herb or a supplement on a daily basis make sure that your physician is aware of it. Get advice from a Doctor who utilizes these disrespected drugs on what to take and how much to take. Make sure there are no conflicts with other medications that you are taking and educate yourself on the possible side effects of those herbs. Have the herbs you are taking compounded by an expert or, if you buy over the counter herbs, buy only quality herbs that bear the USP symbol on the front of the label. Be aware that herbs expire the same way that formulated drugs do. If you are admitted to the hospital and are taking herbs make sure that ALL of the supplements you take are listed on your medication list even if it means repeating it several times. And be aware that most hospitals in the United States do not respect nor provide herbs and supplements to their patients. If you are being treated by a physician outside of the hospital who utilizes herbs in your treatment he will probably need to speak with the in house treating Doctors in order to allow you to continue your regime. If this is the case, be prepared to provide your own preparations.

Provider point: It is your patients' right to know what is going into his or her body. Yes it uses up a lot of your nursing time to have the patient ask what it is every time you give them a pill but let's be honest here: You should have already looked up the medications you need to give and verified them with the Doctors orders. You should already know the action of the drugs you are giving and should be able to just let that knowledge roll off your tongue. That is part of the nursing process that we are all taught while we are in school and, for the safety of your patients, needs to be followed every day. I used to advise my students to state aloud what the medications you are giving are before the patient has to ask. This provides two safety checks. One for you as you listen to yourself say them aloud and a second for you in the patient listening. Plus, if you give a short synopsis of what a medication is for you are providing the patient with the learning aspect of the nursing process and are expanding your own knowledge at the same time that you build confidence and trust with your patient.

Why do hospitals have to serve hospital food? Dietary and the Kitchen

I am going to start this chapter by saying that I have had hospital food that was excellent. It was served to my husband and myself (a guest tray, Thank you) and it was restaurant quality. The main dish was a sirloin tip sauce served over rice. The sauce had fresh mushrooms in it and rice was fluffy. The vegetables on the side were done but still crisp and served with an herb butter that was wonderful. The dinner roll smelled freshly baked and the salad was mixed greens with freshly sliced cucumbers and tomatoes on top. That meal was served to us in a hospital in New Jersey during a two day stay for an emergency situation over 4 years ago. We both still remember it and are both still amazed that it was hospital food. Every other meal we were served there was equally scrumptious. The classic breakfast tray was served with fresh melon on the side and the eggs were fluffy and aromatic with herbs. The sad part of this is that it was so unusual to find quality like that in a hospital setting that we still remember it.

So what made that hospital kitchen different? My guess is that hospital had actually hired a Chef to serve their customers. They obviously cared about their patients. This was also a hospital that provided a decent cot for patient advocates to sleep on and private rooms. It is medium sized hospital, privately managed with staff that was polite without being intrusive and obviously happy to be working there. I am not sure which came first, the quality or the happy staff but it was very refreshing to see that one hospital could have the whole package. The truth be told I am not sure we would remember it in such a positive light if it were not for the fantastic food. When you are trapped in a 12 x 12 room for 24 hours a day the simple pleasures of life become a major focus.

To the opposite end of the spectrum, my husband was once served a plate which contained baked fish, instant mashed potatoes, creamed corn, and some kind of a white pudding. The smell from the fish was so obnoxious that as soon as the lid was lifted from the tray I took it out into the hallway and left it at the nurses' station. My husband was listed as being on a "regular diet"; a hospital term for normal food. Not only did the food stink, the entire serving was white or off white. There was nothing appetizing about it. Now, serving that type of food to someone who is already sick and not really interested in eating defeats a general rule of healing, that being the necessity to provide the body with calories and nutrients needed for the healing you are hoping to obtain. What did I do in this situation? First I went down stairs to the cafeteria to see if the food they sold was any more appetizing. When it was not I took the car keys and went shopping for foods that would entice my husband to eat. That is not a practice that is encouraged by hospital staff.

During a hospital stay the staff keeps track of the amount of food and fluids that patients consume for many reasons. Good nutrition and proper caloric intake are paramount to a positive recovery. Certain complications can be noted by a failure of the patient to eat or drink. One of the indicators for skin breakdown and bed sores is a bad diet. So, once again, why do hospitals serve the quality of food that they do?

One of the excuses is quantity. The kitchen in a hospital has to provide meals for hundreds of people three times a day plus snacks and supplements. It is a huge job. In addition, there is a diversity of requirements for the types of patients they serve. Diabetics are supposed to be served low carbohydrate plates. Some patients require that their food be of a certain consistency to make it easier to swallow. Renal patients have their own requirement of low phosphorous and carefully balanced electrolytes. Cardiac patients get low fat, high fiber diets. At least theoretically.

As a house supervisor I was once called to a diabetic patient's room to hear a complaint about the breakfast tray which contained pancakes with syrup, a biscuit with white gravy, and cream of wheat with sugar and milk. He was angry and I was embarrassed. The tray I reordered for him wasn't much better and I ended up going to the kitchen to obtain protein, in the form of scrambled eggs and turkey sausage, for him. The cooks felt offended by the patients' complaint. Fortunately, this hospital employed a part-time Chef who was semi-retired from working in a restaurant. Instead of being offended, he worked with the staff, and the in-house nutritionist in providing his staff with basic training in nutrition. This was a hospital that provided good quality food, the staff was simply not trained in the variances of dietary requirements of the different patients.

There is in medicine the desire to control every aspect of a patient's life while they are in the hospital. The thought behind this is to be able to identify the cause of any adverse reaction not expected by the medical professionals. As I said, water and fluid intake are documented in the chart. The amount of food consumed off of the tray is also documented. The body's ability to void the waste created by the intake is also documented. Your admitting diagnosis is responsible for the degree of attention paid to these aspects of your care. Specific diets are ordered by Doctors. (Side note here. Most Medical Doctors receive very little training in the field of nutrition. They trust that the ancillary fields will take care of generally specified nutritional needs and most are unaware of the quality of food their patients receive.)

In defense of the kitchen staff most of the people who work in a hospital kitchen have no medical training and most have only a high school diploma. They are minimum wage workers and they do the best with what they are provided. It is the responsibility of the hospital administration to provide the budget which will allow for a nutritionist or a Chef trained in nutrition to plan meals for the patients. This takes an administration willing to look at the holistic picture of medicine and recognize the importance of comfort for their patients. Recognition needs to be given to the balance between aggressive medicine and making a patient feel comfortable. There are progressive hospitals out there that do this.

I mentioned in an earlier chapter a Midwest hospital that provided a family kitchen on every floor so that the patient's family could bring in comfort foods for their loved one. It was a very satisfying solution for many of the patients and their families. The patients received the type of food that their bodies were used to, the families were proud to be part of the healing process, the staff were not inundated with complaints, and the amount of wasted food was greatly decreased. It did require that the nurses have more interaction with the families to evaluate and document the quality and quantity of food the patient received but that too was a positive interaction between staff and families. A nutritionist was available for consultation with families who wished to provide their loved ones with home cooking but needed education on healthy foods.

In my years of hospital work I have also heard the argument that it is a liability to allow patients to provide their own food. While that may be true in some instances, I believe the benefits to be gained from the positive attitude resulting from a good meal far outweighs the risks. If you are unhappy with the quality or type of food that you are receiving talk to your Nurse. Ask her what type of diet the Doctor ordered for you. If it is something you don't understand, ask why that type of diet was ordered. If it still does not make sense to you ask her if the type of diet ordered for you can be changed. If you are still displeased talk to the Doctor.   Tell them you are unhappy with the diet and ask them to change it.

Your Doctor can also order in the chart that your food be brought in from outside the hospital. This is especially an important note to address if you have dietary restrictions for personal reasons such as religious beliefs or allergy problems. Hospitals are not equipped to deal with patient specific orders. Notify your nurse that you are doing this and expect some argument. Nurses are trained to be part of the control of the patient's environment but most are aware of the need for improvement in this area of hospital care and will work with you unless there is a medical reason not to. If you take this route it will be your, or your advocates, responsibility to make sure that you are eating things that assist your body in the healing process. In other words, don't take this as an excuse to eat hamburgers and hot dogs for your entire stay. Potato chips and milk shakes are not nutritionally balanced food.

Please bear in mind that your health comes first while you are in the hospital. Your Doctor may be trying to remove salt from your diet or to control your sugar intake to help improve a medical condition. You do have the right to know and understand why your diet is restricted if it is. A specifically ordered diet is part of the medical treatment and as we already discussed, you have a guaranteed right under the law to understand ALL of your medical treatment. If the restrictions are for a medical reason try to work with the staff. Hopefully you won't be in the hospital for too long and you can indulge when you return home. And you can always ask for supplemental nutrition while in the hospital such prepackaged protein shakes if you find the food not to your liking.

If you have been admitted to the hospital with a diagnosis that can be altered by what you eat such as diabetes, heart problems, renal failure or are on medications that will restrict your diet you can also request that you be given education on how to eat healthy once you arrive home. Your nurse should offer that information to you prior to discharge.

If you have an advocate staying with you they will, in most instances, be responsible for their own food. Some hospitals offer guest trays to families, most do not. Have your advocate ask what hours the cafeteria is open so that they can find their own sustenance. Do not expect or ask the hospital to provide service for them unless it is offered. The hospital's responsibility is to you, not your advocate, and you want them to be happy that you have someone staying with you. Most hospital food is inexpensive in the cafeteria as much of the staff eat there. Most all now have a salad or soup bar which is very affordable. Do not expect free anything for your advocate. Hospitals are businesses. A good advocate will come prepared with bottled water and protein bars.

I believe that with the hospital industries recognition of the need for providing comfort measures for their patients the quality of food will be addressed. Hospitals are in competition for your business and this is just another way to keep people happy. I recently saw a sign up in one hospital offering senior citizens meals at a 50% discount. A great public service was being provided and it kept that hospital forefront in the minds of the senior citizens in the community. And, of course, the quality of the food has to be good if you are going to offer it to the community.

"Who was that masked man?" or Doctors, Nurses, and other things that go bump in the night

One of the biggest shortcomings by hospital personnel that I have found over the years is the failure of staff to introduce themselves properly. As professionals that work in a very exclusionary business we tend to think that the general public knows as much about our job descriptions and identities as we do. Immersed in the society of the medical center we fail to understand the intimidation that the labyrinth of specialties and personnel a patient must work through to find their path to good health. And to make matters worse, we all dress the same! People that work in the hospital may understand the subtle difference between green scrubs for surgery staff and blue for floor nurses but the general public does not. And even if we give them a map of the colors that the different departments are wearing, there is still the failure to identify the Surgeon from the anesthesiologist from the surgical radiology tech, from the nurse, etc.

There remains the culture centric thought that people know the difference between the jobs that the anesthesiologist and the scrub nurse perform. The solution to this problem would seem quite simple from the outside; staff should introduce themselves. Not once but every time they provide care to a patient. As care givers we seemingly forget that the people that we are treating are not only in a stressed situation, physically impaired, and also probably medicated. We all dress the same and in most facilities hair has to be worn groomed, so we look similar even if our features are very different.

Staff should be encouraged to explain briefly their role in the continuation of a patients care daily. While this is usually part of the training, it is a not something that most care givers take the time to do as they take for granted that everyone knows what a nurse does.

One of the ways that hospitals have addressed this issue is with 'white boards' where they list things like 'Nurse', 'Nursing Assistant', 'Charge Nurse', 'Case Manager', and 'Respiratory' with corresponding names of staff but without explaining the function of those positions. The general public, as a whole, does not understand the differences in education and practice between a Certified Nursing Assistant and a Nurse.

Another step that some of the larger medical facilities have taken to help with identifying different employees is to dress different staff in different colored scrubs. With the loss of the iconic nursing cap and after years of having patients ask housekeepers and cafeteria workers who also are dressed in scrubs, for advice on their medical care or for another pain pill, these facilities have taken to dressing the nurses in one color, usually royal blue, and ancillary personal in others. This helps somewhat if the course of your action is explained to the patient. However, it remains in the patient's best interest to have staff trained not only to introduce themselves when they enter the room but also give a very brief synopsis of the function they will perform. "Hi. I'm Linda. I will be your nurse today. I will bring you your medications and help with organizing your care. If you need anything you should ask to speak to me as I am the one who knows what the Doctor wants you to have and what we hope to accomplish for you during your stay here." Sounds simple. It simply doesn't happen. Nurses that do introduce themselves say things such as "I'm your primary nurse." Without stopping to realize that 'Primary nurse' is not a term used by the general public and has no assigned definition to it.

It is true that almost all hospitals require staff to wear name tags. These are those little pieces of plastic that flip around happily on a stretchy string effectively hiding the name and function of the provider at least 50% of the time. While in the future evolution of the hospital setting I believe we will find a viable solution to the identity problem right now it remains a mystery, so I will attempt to help with the basic identification of those people who keep coming into your room.

Let's start with the Doctors.   Medicine is a huge and involved art of science. The number of Doctors that you will be seeing during your stay is exponential to the number of diagnosis on your admission chart. Very rarely will you only be seeing your personal physician.   But, for lack of any other reason than chance, we will start here.

Your primary care physician. He or she attended college for four years before applying to and being admitted to a medical school. Medical school includes two years of book learning and lectures plus two years of clinical rotations where students learn how to interact with real life patients. After this training Doctors have to take 'Boards' which is a fancy way of saying they have to take a test to determine if they have learned enough to be considered a Doctor. If they pass the "Boards" they are technically Doctors but they are not finished with their training yet. Now they have to spend two or three years doing an internship. Internship is further exposure to patients in various settings. Specialties can be chosen at this juncture or Doctors can continue to pursue general medical studies. Following this Internship Doctors are free to enter practice however most physicians will spend an additional two to four years in a Residency which is specialized training. The range of these is extensive but most physicians who work as primary care Doctors specialized in either Family practice or Internal medicine. Specialists are not limited to their specialty but can chose to serve as primary care physicians.

Your Doctor works for you. Ask what they were trained in. This is important as Doctors tend to focus their care on what their training was in. Just to confuse matters further there are also M.D.'s which stands for Medical Doctor, and D.O. which is a Doctor of Osteopathy. The training between these two is basically the same although a D.O. has more training in the bone structure and manipulation of bone structure. There is little difference in the basic training here and one should not be considered more suited to primary care than the other.

Doctors that serve as personal or primary care physicians usually have a Doctor's Office where you can make an appointment to be seen. They follow your care and help with the coordination of any of the specialty physicians you may require. Medicine is a huge field and very involved. There is no Doctor that knows it all and if your Doctor tells you he does you should probably look for a new Doctor. A good primary care physician will not only refer you to the appropriate specialist but will make sure that the specialist you see is a good one. Your primary care Doctor should be sent copies of tests ordered by specialists as, like I said, it is their job to coordinate the care you need. Your primary Doctor should also be kept advised of any medications that another Doctor orders for you. This is so he or she can make sure there are no problems with interaction of medications although filling all prescriptions at the same pharmacy will allow a licensed Pharmacist to review these for you.

While a Pharmacist is not a Medical Doctor they do have the same years of training that M.D.s do specializing in the chemistry of medications and their effects on the body, so as far as medicines are concerned this is your best bet. All hospitals have Pharmacists on staff to prepare your medications, reconcile your home medications with the drugs that the admitting Doctor wants you to take while you are in the hospital, and make sure they are delivered safely. If you have an adverse reaction to a medication or the wrong medication is administered you will meet this person. While they are usually very busy providing medications for an entire hospital full of patients 24 hours a day, they are caring people who will take the time to address any concerns about your medicines that you cannot satisfy by talking to your Nurse or your Doctor.

Not all primary physicians, nor all specialists for that matter, will have hospital privileges. Hospital privileges are granted by the hospital on the recommendation of the Medical Staff.   These are based generally on back ground checks that include verifying graduation from an accredited medical school, an approved residency, and that the medical license of the physician is in good standing. There is also a consideration as to the need of the hospital and the public they serve. There is no need to have 15 OB's on staff in a geriatric community in South Florida. Sometimes these decisions can be very politically biased since Doctors are still people and have the same emotional responses as the rest of us.

If your primary care physician does not have privileges at a hospital that you are admitted to he cannot give orders for the course of your treatment directly to the hospital staff. He can, however, work through the Hospitalist to help guide your care.

What is a Hospitalist? A hospitalist is a relatively new specialty in which a Doctor treats patients currently in the hospital. There are good and bad aspects to the idea of a Hospitalist. On the good side, there is always a Doctor available in the Hospital, they don't have to be called at the office or tracked down at home to get orders for the Tylenol you need for your headache. It also guarantees that you will see a Doctor every day that you are in the hospital. Unfortunately, the Doctor you see will not know your medical history the way that your primary care Doctor does nor will he have the same personal interest in your care. Hospitalist care is based on the current diagnosis and what is in your chart. Also, these Doctors are notoriously overworked. They are treating every patient currently in the hospital. Because of that they have a tendency to work on protocols that dictate the treatment path of specific diagnosis. Since every human body is different, this is not always in the best interest of the patient. If new medications or treatments are added to your routine, ask why. If tests are ordered, ask why.

In some hospitals the Hospitalists maintain all the in-house care even if your primary care physician has privileges. One of the questions you should ask when choosing a primary care physician should be whether or not they will retain your care if you are admitted to a hospital.

Specialists. This is a huge category and I won't attempt to cover all of them. A definition of Physician specialties and what they do for you could fill a book all on its own. If a specialist is assigned to your care, ask them what they do. Don't be intimidated by the Doctor title. It is your body and you have a right to know who is looking at it and why. I once had a patient who had been seeing an Oncologist (a cancer specialist) for two weeks before he happened to ask a nurse why that Doctor was seeing him and what all the new medications were for. It was not a good way to find out he had cancer and yet the staff just assumed that he would know that an Oncologist treats people with cancer.

Human nature being what it is, it is not unusual for people to want to just hand over their care to the powers that be. That is NEVER a good idea. Anyway, I digress, back to specialists. I will try to cover the most common specialties seen in a hospital setting.

Emergency Doctors. Emergency medicine did not used to be a specialty. It was a job that was covered by whatever physician happened to be on call or wanted the extra hours or work. It was finally recognized as the specialty that it is in the early 1970's. As someone who has an extensive personal history of working in emergency settings I have a profound respect for these physicians. These doctors are amazing at taking collections of ambiguous symptoms from people they have never met before, ordering appropriate tests, finding diagnoses, and prescribing treatment paths. I have watched emergency physicians run two codes at the same time while maintaining a handle on every other patient in their emergency departments. They determine who will be admitted from the emergency department and are responsible for convincing the admitting Doctor, whether that be your primary care Doctor or a Hospitalist, that they truly believe you need to be treated in the hospital. If you are sent home they will advise you of your course of action and refer you to appropriate follow-up care.

Surgeons. This is one of those specialties where there are multiple subspecialties. General surgeons do general surgery like taking out your appendix. Orthopedic surgeons work on repairing bones. Thoracic surgeons operate on the organs and vasculature of the inside of the chest. Vascular surgeons work on veins and arteries. This is also one of those specialties where you want to request the sub-specialist. These guys are going into your insides with sharp implements. You want the one that has cut on similar parts many times over. Surgeons consider themselves to be one of the elite specialties in medicine. They can be very exacting (a good thing while they are digging around in your innards) and demanding. In fact there is a joke in medicine that the only difference between God and a Surgeon is that God doesn't think he is a

Surgeon. Funny but also definitely an attitude you want from this specialty unless you are the nurse they are giving orders too.

Anesthesiologists. These are the Doctors who maintain the delicate balance between unconsciousness and death while you are having surgery. Most of the medications that are given during an operation can also kill you if this delicate balance is not managed. They watch your breathing (or make sure it is done for you), your blood pressure, heart rate, and make sure you stay unconscious and don't feel the pain while the surgeon does his magic.   You will probably only meet this specialist once and that will be shortly before your surgery when he or she shows up to ask you questions about allergies to medications or shellfish and family history of reactions to anesthetics. There are also nurses that work in this role who have specialized training in this fine - tuned art. There are quite a few newer anesthetics on the market which have fewer serious side -affects and are easier to reverse than the ones you hear horror stories about. Talk to this person if you are anxious before surgery. It is part of their job to let you know what drug they will be giving to you, the effect they will have on your body, and what to expect afterwards. They won't be able to tell you about your surgery. The surgeon should do that.

Radiologist. This is one of the Doctors that will be involved with your care, you will get a bill from, and yet never see.   This is a Doctor who has specialized in reading x-rays, CT scans, MRI's, and all that other stuff we talked about in the chapter on Radiology. That's all he or she does. Are you wondering why your own physician can't read x-rays? The answer is that he or she probably can but not with the experienced, detailed eye of a radiologist.

Pathologist. Another invisible Doctor who is integral to your care that you will never see. This is the person in the lab who looks at things that either come out of you or are removed from you like urine, blood, or that cyst that they biopsied. He or she is the one who looks at all of that stuff and then lets your Doctor know if there are serious disease processes in play and what they are.

Obstetrician. Usually pared with a double specialty in Gynecology this is a Doctor who specialized in the study of childbirth and all the female parts that go along with that. There are many of these Doctors that are dropping the Obstetrician part of this due to uncontrolled malpractice insurance costs for Doctors who deliver babies.

Psychiatrist. This is a medical Doctor who has extensive training in the study and chemistry of the mind. This is the Doctor you will be referred to if you are found to have a mental problem that may have an underlying physical cause. Severe depression is also something that should be addressed by a Psychiatrist due to their knowledge of the delicate balance in the chemistry of the brain. While Psychiatrists will also talk to you and help you figure out all the ugly stuff that happened to you as a child they should not be confused with Psychologists who focus on cause and effect and are not trained as Medical Doctors.

Neurologist. The structure of the nervous system and brain is the focus of this specialty. You will see this Doctor if you have a stroke, seizures, one of the diseases that affects the nervous system (such as Parkinson's) or any injury to the head or nervous system.

Dermatologist. This is a Doctor who deals with problems with the skin. Although we take it for granted, the skin is actually one of your vital organs. It not only holds everything together for you but it is responsible for the regulation of body temperature, moisture content, and protection of your insides from the myriad of potential damaging and invading threats you deal with every day.

Podiatrist. This is a specialty that focuses on the diseases and injuries of the foot. Podiatrists attend a specialized school to receive their four years of training. That is usually followed by a three year residency program.

Rheumatologist.   These Doctors specialize in treating patients with Arthritis and other rheumatoid diseases. Rheumatoid diseases include any disease that can cause inflammation, swelling and damage to the joints and, sometimes, other organs. This includes auto-immune diseases where your immune system attacks your body.

As I said earlier I could go on and on with the diversity of Doctors that exist out there. There are even specialist that deal with different ages of people and the specialized problems seen in those age groups such as pediatrics and geriatrics. If you think you need a specialist and one has not been assigned to you, ask your primary physician or the hospitalist.

One more thing I need to say about Doctors and that has to do with the hierarchy. Every hospital has a Medical Director who is a physician and heads up regular meetings of the medical staff. If you have problems with your Doctor or the one that treated you in house you can file a complaint with the Medical Director who will review it. Doctors are a rather closed community but they are also very proud of their chosen profession and if there is a problem with one of their numbers they will address it.

It bears repeating that as a general rule the Doctors do not work for the hospital, they are contracted through it usually by a medical group from outside of the hospital. However, complaints against a Doctor can be addressed to the administration of the hospital and they will make sure that it is followed up on through appropriate channels. Medicine has become a competitive field which means that the hospital wants you to choose to go to their facility when you are sick.

Mid-level providers. This is a fairly new field developed to assist overworked physicians. There are two main types of mid-level providers; Nurse Practitioners and Physician Assistants. The main difference between the two is the training and experience they had before going to school to be a mid-level care provider. A Nurse Practitioner or NP is a Registered Nurse who has continued on with her training in nursing school usually to the level of a Master's Degree. She or he usually has years of experience working as a nurse prior to going back to school. A Physicians' Assistant or PA took the same Mid-level training as the NP but probably had little or no medical training or experience prior to the two year course that earned them their credentials. In some states admission to a PA program does not even require a Bachelor degree prior to admission.

Nurses and the nursing field. There are different levels of training for people who provide direct patient care. A CNA is a Certified Nurse Assistant. They are trained in comfort measures for patients and in how to assist Nurses with vital signs and other simple tasks. If your hospital still employs CNA's in spite of budgetary cuts consider yourself lucky as this person is the one who will make sure you get a bath, dinner while it is still hot, and bring you that extra blanket if you are chilled. This is not the person to ask about your medical treatment. The training of this person is usually through a technical school and varies in intensity and quality, but the average training is 6 weeks.

The LVN is a Licensed Vocational Nurse. This is a certificate level nurse who has received about a year of medical training. This level of nursing is slowly being eased out of hospital settings. I have worked with LVN's that were extraordinary in their practice and I would put them up against any RN however, the evolution of the nursing practice demands the extension of education that is involved in that practice. There are programs available that will take LVN's up to the RN level and I strongly advise any LVN who wants to continue her practice to apply to one of these programs even if it means taking extra college courses to qualify. An in depth understanding of the patho/physiology of the human body is mandatory to providing quality nursing care in this era of fast paced medical care.

RN stands for Registered Nurse. At a minimum this is two-years of training in a nursing school. Like the LVN's the certificate level RN is rapidly being phased out. Hospitals want the RN's with degrees. The minimum training for an RN with a degree is an Associate's Degree that takes 3 to 4 years to complete including all the pre-requisites of the programs and completion of a program specifically addressing the art of nursing. These nurses have training in anatomy, physiology, nutrition, chemistry, pharmacology, and patient care. Most of the nurses you meet out there will hold an ADN degree which is an Associate Degree in Nursing. Most also hold an AS degree which is an Associate of Science although an AA degree, Associate of Arts, is also common. An RN with a bachelor degree has basically the same training in patient care but will have more training in administrative organization.

There are also a myriad of training levels for nurses after graduation. NP means Nurse Practitioner and is a master degree in nursing with training to work independently under the direction of a physician as previously stated. Nursing instructors usually have Master's degree with a focus on administration or education as do most Hospital Nursing Administrators. There is also a Doctorate of Nursing available in both administration and clinical studies. Nursing is an evolving field that will continue to change along with our growing and aging population. The more complicated medicine becomes the greater the need will be for nurses to help orchestrate and manage patient care.

In addition to the above basic levels of training most Nurses continue their education and careers with specialized education. Nursing

144

schools are pretty basic in what they teach. Nurses that choose to work in specialized departments can get accreditation (which also goes along with a higher level of pay) by taking additional training classes. ICU nurses take Critical care classes. Emergency Room nurses take training that is specific to emergency situations. Most of those little letters following a nurse's name on her badge represent the specialized credentials she or he has chosen to pursue.

There are also many hospital administration that require a degree in nursing. Chief among these is the Director of Nursing. This is a nurse with an advanced degree who oversees the Nurses that work in the hospital. If you have a problem with a nurse on the staff at a hospital this is her ultimate boss. There is a chain of command that is followed from the patient care nurse to reach the Director of Nursing which depends primarily on the size of the hospital but she or he is at the top of that chain. This person is responsible for seeing that only qualified Licensed Nurses practice in the facility, that their level of training is adequate to the needs of the community and that the staff is provided with training to keep them competent in the evolving world of hospital medicine.   She is ultimately responsible for the behavior of her nurses.

That brings us to chain of command in the nursing community. If you have a complaint with a nurse your first step is to address it with the Charge Nurse on the floor. If you do not find regress there your next step is usually the head of the department that the nurse works in. In the larger hospitals the next in the chain of command is a floor supervisor followed by the house supervisor. Nurses are generally caring, loving people who got into this profession because they wanted to make a difference in the world. You will occasionally find a cranky one, or an over worked one, or simply someone who chose the wrong profession but somewhere in this chain someone will listen to you.   And chances are if you encountered a nurse who is rude or seems uncaring, her supervisor is already aware of the problem.

There are two other positions that are traditionally filled by Registered Nurses that you will meet in the course of your stay. The first is a Case Manager. This person is responsible for making sure that you are receiving all the services that you require from the hospital during your stay. She is also very knowledgeable in hospital charges and insurance payments. This is the person who will figure out how things should be documented in order to provide you with the best return on your medical insurance bill.

Sometimes combined with the above mentioned position, a Discharge Planner is a nurse who will make sure that you have all the services that you need when you are discharged from the hospital. If the Doctor discharges you but wants you to continue with Oxygen at home, this is the person who will arrange for it to be delivered before you get home. She can assist you with getting home health care if you need it, set you up with a primary care physician if you don't have one, and even help you find a ride home.

Another adjunct to the hospital setting which are under-appreciated are the Physical Therapists. These people usually carry a Bachelor's Degree or higher specializing in the physical form and function of the support system for the body. If you have trouble getting out of bed or are a little wobbly on your feet after an extended illness these people are the ones that show up at your bedside with devices to assist you in your mechanical physical recovery. They will teach you how to retrain weak muscles and make sure that you know how to avoid falling until you are back to your prime state. Working with case managers they will make sure that you have the necessary tools upon your release to help you be as self-sufficient as possible. Physical Therapists also work outside of the hospital setting in rehab units and private gyms that assist people recover function lost as a result of illness or injury. Ask them to provide written copies of the exercises they feel you need on your discharge and do not underestimate the importance of what they teach you. They are a major step on your way to recovering full function.

Respiratory Therapists, or RT's, usually have an Associate's Degree. Their training is highly focused on airway management and disease process that affect the lungs. Like RN's they can continue on with their studies and advance their careers. This is someone you will see quite frequently if you have breathing problems. Asthma, bronchitis, COPD, and CHF are just some of the conditions they will help to treat. There was a move a few years ago by hospital administrators to reduce the hours of Respiratory therapists as a cost cutting device. It didn't last long. One of the things most people are really fond of is the ability to breath.

Lab technicians also require an Associate degree in order to practice although there are still certificate level programs available for people with a documented medical background. Be aware that the person that draws your blood is not necessarily a Lab Technician. That person was probably a Phlebotomist. A phlebotomist is someone who is trained to draw blood and put it in tubes. Training for that certification is usually 6 weeks. Lab Technicians, because of the higher level of education and thus a higher rate of pay are usually utilized in the laboratory itself. The people that travel around with the little carts are usually phlebotomists but be assured that they are very good at sticking needles into veins. They get LOTS of practice.

Radiology Technicians are the people who take x-rays of you. This is a position that is slowly evolving with medicine. Right now the position requires, at a minimum, a two year training program that is not degreed but a certificate level. In 2015 an Associate's Degree will be required to take the exam for the certification to practice. With all the advancement in this branch of medicine and the level of technology they use it is really no surprise.

In addition to all of these people the hospital is staffed with support personnel such as house keepers, registration clerks, and kitchen helpers. All of these people have had at least a minimum of training in first aid and interacting with patients although they are not the ones to address your medical questions or complaints to.

Housekeepers are trained in special cleaning methods that address some of the nasty germs that breed in hospitals. There are degreed programs in maintenance of hospitals and the head of these departments usually have this education unless you are in a smaller community hospital. Hospitals would cease to function without these people. The germs would overtake them and we would all die of nasty infections. I once knew a nursing instructor who had a question on her final which stated "What is the first name of the Housekeeper on your shift?" The question carried a high enough point score that it could make you or break you on the final and taught a very important lesson to more than one aspiring nurse.

Of course, there are maintenance people who will come to your room to do any repairs that are needed to the non-medical equipment such as doors, windows, lights, beds, plumbing, etc. They will even adjust the temperature in your room for you if you request.

The kitchen staff is usually over seen by a Nutritionist. This is a degreed position, usually 4 years, which addresses the nutritional needs of certain types of patients. You will probably during your stay receive a visit from the nutritionist. She or he will ask you about your likes, dislikes, and address your nutritional needs. This person can provide you with educational insight into specific diet types such as the diabetic diet. He or she will be working in conjuncture with the Kitchen manager and the kitchen staff to provide you with food while you are staying in the hospital. If you have specific likes or dislikes make sure you tell them when they make rounds to collect menus. They will attempt to make this important aspect of your stay acceptable to you. Definitely make sure that you tell both them and the nurse if you have any food allergies.

Registration clerks are the people who greet you when you first come into the hospital. This position usually requires a high school degree at a minimum, typing and computer skills, plus really good people skills. These are the people who set the initial tone for your visit to the hospital. The good ones will give you that smile and relaxed demeanor which is very reassuring when you're being admitted to the hospital.

In addition to all the people you will meet and interact with there are huge numbers of people who work behind the scenes to keep the hospital functioning. There are medical record clerks who make sure your documents are safe and filed so that they are easily accessed if future need dictates. They will also make sure that your insurance company gets the records they need so that they can pay your bill.

There also exists another entire indispensable group of people working in a department called Central Supply. These are the people who order, catalog, store and deliver to different department all of the supplies needed by staff and patients over the course of a day. These people make sure that there are tissues in your room as well as Normal Saline for your IV. If the floor runs out of a special supply these people will order it and then deliver it to the floor.

The number of hospitals that have their own laundry facilities has decreased over the past decades. There was a time when it was the duty of the nursing staff to not only wash the sheets from the bed but also to sharpen the needles for reuse. Those days are long gone. The emergence of frightening new bacteria strains and cross contamination between patients has turned hospital laundry into a specialty field. Cleaning agents that will kill all of those bacteria and viruses and temperatures hot enough to sterilize linen are mandatory. Disposal of the chemical and waste laden result of this is a huge environmental concern.

Some hospitals also employ people under a generalized title of technician. This can be preceded by defining categories such as Transportation technician. Many ED's employ Emergency Medical Technicians (EMT's) in their emergency departments to help with basic chores. EMT's, however, do have training of at least 6 weeks in care of people in emergency situations. Some hospitals also employ Paramedics in this role. Paramedics have intensive training which lasts from two to four years in emergency medicine. If you came to the hospital in an ambulance chances are you had a team of one Paramedic and one EMT to assist. Fire fighters are usually trained as EMT's.

So those are the people that work in the hospital that are in direct contact with patients. If I have forgotten anyone, I apologize profusely as hospitals function only due to the team work between all the various parties employed there. The next chapter will contain more information on the administration in the hospital. These are the people who you will probably never see but are there to assure that everything works the way it is supposed to.

Hospital Administrators and the chain of command

There are a lot of things that can go wrong in a hospital. It is a huge building full of people (most of them type A personalities) and anytime you find large groups of people that have to communicate to obtain a goal, you will find problems developing. So let us do a little triage here when it comes to problems in a hospital. We will start with the medical side of it. You are in the hospital because you are sick or injured. Something is seriously enough wrong with your body that you are lying in that uncomfortable bed with people assigned to care for you. Something is not feeling right. What do you do?

Frighteningly, doing a quick internet search on hospital chain of command will produce dozens of web sites most of which address nurses. These web sites all provide information for the nurse on how to document her care of her patient and what steps to take to avoid 'getting in trouble' when something goes wrong. The really scary part here is that YOU, the patient, are the 'something that could go wrong." Having your nurse know how to document that she knew something was wrong so that she does not get into trouble is not going to do you or your health any good. So when do you, as a patient, if you feel that something is wrong, call for help? Maybe your symptoms are worse or you have new symptoms that you didn't have before you came in. Should you worry about that prickly rash that is spreading over your belly?

This is really very basic medicine here. That is your body that you are living in. You have owned it and resided in it for your whole life. If you have a feeling that something is wrong, you owe it to yourself to get it checked out. In fact, most of the best practitioners that I know teach new students that the best way to find out what is wrong with a patient is to talk to them. People know when something is wrong with them. Yes, things seem worse when you are stressed, or tired, but you also know your body better than anyone else. If you are concerned about something unusual that is happening to it, call someone to check it out.

Now the challenge: If you are already in the hospital and you suspect that something is going wrong who do you call? Well, first, your nurse. She is the one responsible for your well-being while you are assigned to her care. If she is good at her job she will listen to you. Even if she is not that good at her job but had adequate training, she will listen to you. (Remember all those web sites we just talked about that were telling nurses how to stay out of trouble?) Even if you are frightened by what is happening, speak clearly and as calmly as you can when you describe your new symptom. Your nurse should look at the part of your body that is giving you trouble and check your vital signs to look for changes. She should ask you questions that remind you of all those questions you were asked when you first came into the hospital. "When did it start?" "On a scale of one to ten, how bad is it?" "Have you had this symptom before?"

After she examines you and checks your vital signs (blood pressure, heart rate, etc.) she will advise you on what she feels is going on. Now remember that this person is a trained professional. They went to school for many years to learn about things that can go wrong with the human body. He or she cares for a large number of people every year. Listen to her. She may have seen the problem that you are having before and know exactly what to do for you to make you better.   If you are not comfortable with what she is telling you, tell her that. Nicely. If this is a good competent nurse, they will either call your Doctor to advise him of your new symptom or have one of the nursing supervisors come in to look at you.

If he or she calls for the immediate supervisor it will be the floor charge nurse. Almost all hospital units are overseen by one nurse who supervises and helps out the other nurses on the floor. She is usually a more experienced nurse with very good people skills. Repeat to her what you told your other nurse.   Tell her your concerns. This is not a time to complain that your first nurse did not know what to do. She knows that. That is why she is in the room with you. Stay focused on your problem no matter how frustrating this gets. The charge nurse should examine you and talk to you, probably making you repeat everything you just told the other nurse. Then she will either address the problem with you or if she doesn't' know what to do, she will call the Doctor.

This is not the time to get angry or to let your frustration show. Nurses are human beings and if you start addressing them in an aggressive manner you will eventually push the wrong button. That means that your problem is not going to be addressed with the same concern as if you had asked politely. Threatening to "sue the hospital" if you don't see the doctor immediately will get you exactly nowhere. First of all, the nurses have no control over the Doctors and second of all, they have all heard that threat a thousand times before. Hospitals are frustrating places. They know that. They work there. Try to be patient (no pun intended).

Most medical problems in hospitals are resolved or recognized with these few basic steps. However, there are times when patients are not listened to or are ignored due to communication problems (see above), understaffing, tired staff, or burned-out nurses. Sometimes Doctors can't be reached in an expedient manner. Anytime there are people involved there is room for error.

If your problem is still not resolved what do you do? You keep trying. Once again, this is your body. You know it better than anyone in that hospital because you live in it. If they cannot help you resolve the problem that you having medically you owe it to yourself to pursue it. Hopefully, you have an advocate with you that can serve as your cheerleader here but when the staff asks you questions about what is going on, you should be the one to respond to the questions, not your advocate.

If the charge nurse cannot help you and your Doctor does not respond, ask to speak to a floor manager or a House Supervisor. Floor managers are administratively trained nurses that have worked their way up to a position where they supervise a hospital unit. They normally have special training and experience in the type of medicine that is practiced on the floor they manage. However, Nursing Managers usually only work weekday hours: Monday through Friday 8:00 to 5:00. Hours vary according to the size of the hospital and the type of supervision provided by the Manager.

Your other option here is the House Supervisor. This is a nurse who is cross -trained in every department of the hospital and usually has an extensive history of patient care experience. She is also responsible for the smooth running of the hospital and the safety of her staff so he or she should be very responsive to your needs. You can ask your nurse to page the House Supervisor or if you are meeting resistance in the chain of command, you can use your bedside phone to call the operator and ask them to page the Supervisor to your room.

Another option, at this level is a specially trained team who can reassess a patient (examine you fully) at the request of the patient or the nurse. These teams are becoming quite popular as they save lives, hospital hours, and staff frustration by identifying deteriorating patient medical conditions before they become an emergency. Your hospital will have notified you upon your admission if they have such a team available. In most facilities that have organized such teams they are referred to as Rapid Response Teams. It you don't remember what they said in all that paperwork we discussed earlier, ask your nurse if they have such a team. They will come to your room and completely reevaluate you. If you need extra treatment they will see that you get it. These teams usually work on protocols set by the hospital that let them start treatments on patients without contacting the physician first. They will, of course, notify your physician of any and all changes in your condition that they identify and report to him or her any steps they have taken to solve the problem. Such teams usually consist of an ICU nurse, an emergency nurse, a respiratory therapist and (sometimes) a physicians' assistant or a Nurse practitioner. Once again you will need to repeat all of the information that you have already provided to your staff nurse and her supervisor. Being asked your Name and Birthdate is standard safety practice and if it doesn't happen enough to be really annoying you should be concerned.

If there is no team and you are still not satisfied that your condition is being addressed properly, ask to talk to the Doctor directly. This may be your physician or the hospitalist depending on your hospital policy. A private call to your Doctor's office can stimulate concern in the hospital if your doctor's office is personal in their approach to the care of their own patients.

Your next step is to move on up the chain of command. Remember that at this point we are addressing problems with your body, a change in your medical condition that you feel is not getting enough concern. I do not want you calling all the way up the chain of command because the TV in your room does not get 35 channels or they served you orange Jell-O when you requested pudding. (Yes, I have been called to patients rooms to address both of those problems) The key to getting attention in a hospital when you feel you need it is to be the squeaky wheel (which gets the oil it needs), not the charging bull (which people avoid).

If you have listed your concerns for your well- being with all of the above and still have not received some type of resolution then your next step is to call the office of the Director of Nurses or the Chief Nurse Administrator. Most of the time just asking for the number for this office will get action and attention from the nursing staff as this is their ultimate boss. He or she is responsible for the actions of all of the nursing staff that works within that hospital. This is a Registered Nurse that has worked her way up the ladder to the position of ultimate authority when it comes to nursing staff within the hospital. She not only has patient care training but is politically motivated to keep you, the customer, happy with her staff.

I should also note here that since the implementation of the HCAHPS (Hospital Consumer Assessment of Healthcare Providers and Systems) survey, full hospital reimbursement can be withheld if the public satisfactions scores are too low.   I will address this more in the chapter on discharge.

Every hospital has a different line up of administrators.   The Director of Nurses goes by many different titles. She can be listed as The Director of Nursing, the Chief Nurse Administrator, the Vice-President of Patient Care Services; the list goes on. Titles vary but the position remains the same. This is the top of the nursing chain. That does not mean the top of the Administrative Chain of the Hospital. The Director of Nurses works for the Chief Executive Officer of the Hospital who works for the board of Directors.

There is quite a variance in hospitals as to how the chain of command is set up but these positions are usually standard. Medical degrees or training is not required for most of the positions that exist over the Director of Nurses so they will not be able to answer your medical questions. Most hospital administrators are very proud of the hospitals they represent. They can and will respond if you have concerns that are not being answered.

"I really just want to go home now" Which means Discharge planning

Discharge planning is supposed to start the minute you are admitted to the hospital. The social worker or Registered Nurse that is responsible for this task and holds the title of Discharge Planner should be reviewing your medical information and financial situation daily. They usually make rounds with the hospital team during the day to hear updated information about the condition, progress, and prognosis for every patient in house. I say usually because that is in a perfect world. Things happen, especially in the larger institutions with large numbers of patients.

Following your basic progression through the medical maze allows discharge planners to, quite simply, have a plan for you when you are released from the hospital. Sometimes this is a simple plan; you go home with your loved ones and continue your life. Sometimes it is more complicated: Do you need someone to help you cope with daily living when you get home? Do you need special medical supplies waiting for your arrival back home? The discharge planner is the one responsible for making sure that these things are in place when the Doctor decides it is OK for you to be released from the hospital.

Sometimes, especially these days, being released from the hospital does not mean you are able to take care of yourself again just yet. Insurance (Medicare included) only allows for a certain number of paid days in the hospital depending on your medical diagnosis. Predetermining the number of days in the hospital required by every individual based on the diagnosis and recovery of other unknown strangers is not a good idea since everybody is different but that is the way it is done. A good hospital staff can work around this and sometimes keep you longer than dictated by your primary diagnosis but usually the numbers stand. If you are delayed in your recovery a discharge planner can arrange for you to be moved to a sub-acute care facility such as a nursing home. They can also arrange for a nurse to come into your home and assist you with medical procedures that are still required. They can even arrange, in some instances, for you to have someone come into your home and help with daily living chores, such as bathing and housework. The Planner will look at your needs and check to make sure which alternative will best fit with your available insurance coverage and financial state. She will also have a list of outside resources that may be available for you such as organizations which help provide meals in your home or services.

It is in the best interest of the hospital to make sure that you continue on your path to good health once released as a relapse that leads to a readmission within 30 days of discharge is not usually covered by insurance and the hospital will be held liable. (This is also true of any injuries or infections that you acquire while you are in the hospital.) So every effort is made to make sure that you will have adequate care until you fully recover.

There are, of course, people that fall through the cracks. I recently learned that a friend of a family member was released early from a local hospital and ended up living in an uninsulated garage that had been approved by the state for post hospital care. The people running the "home" were not interested in patient care issues, they were in it for the money paid by the state. He ate canned sausages and junk food. The problem was that he had no private insurance and the public assistance available to him was limited by his diagnosis. When the Discharge Planner was questioned she explained that because his situation was unusual it was the garage or a homeless shelter. She was as frustrated by the situation as the patient but the financial aspects were beyond her control.

The point being that the Discharge Planner is not a miracle worker but will do as much as they can to see that you have what is needed after your discharge. In most cases there are also outside entities available to assist. And this is another place where a good patient advocate can be priceless. Chances are you will still not be feeling very well on your discharge from the hospital. Most people just want to go home and sleep in the quiet of their own bed after nights of hospital noise. But pay close attention to this Planner when they come to speak with you prior to discharge. Ask questions. Don't refuse any services until you have had time to think about it and discuss it with your advocate.

If no one comes into your room and questions you about your care when you are released, ask your nurse. In some facilities the necessity for discharge planning is made based on the notes made by your Doctor and Nurse. Once again, this is an area where you need to be asking a lot of questions especially if you are going home disabled. Tell the nurse if you have concerns about caring for yourself or special adjustments that need to be made. Ask if there is a Discharge Planner available to answer your questions and provide you with information of services that will be available to you.

When you do get home from your hospital you may receive a "Patient Satisfaction Survey". This is not just your hospital trying to find out if they kept you happy. This is a national survey that was first implemented in 2002 and is gradually growing in power. In fact since 2007 some payment reimbursement to hospitals can be reduced if the hospitals do not meet with certain levels of satisfaction. Federally funded, the HCAHPS collects data from randomly selected patients within 6 weeks of discharge from the hospital. This survey addresses several categories of patient satisfaction during their stay including hospital cleanliness, staff communication, pain control, responsiveness, and communication related to medications and discharge planning. You will also be asked to rate the hospital and whether or not you would recommend it to family or friends. If you hear staff talking about H-cap scores this is what they mean. This is a fascinating development in the control of the quality of healthcare in this country and it will be exciting to see where it leads. If you would like more information on this survey, the federal requirements for it, and basic information about how it developed you can visit the website: www.hcahpsonline.org. If you would like information about the hospital you are staying in and how it compares nationally and on a state wide level you can look it up at:www.hospitalcompare.hhs.gov . If you are one of the people chosen to take this survey, please take the few minutes it requires to complete it. And be honest as you take it. Federal interest in the improvement in the quality of your hospital stay is a huge improvement from the past.

A Final Word

Hospitals are a necessary part of our modern society. They allow people suffering from illness and/or injury to be cared for in a central setting complete with the technology needed to evaluate and treat most medical problems. The financial/business end of the hospital experience has grown by leaps and bounds creating huge conglomerates in which remaining a name with the face becomes a challenge to both staff and patients. Problems have been created by the sheer magnitude of the institutes we have created. The evolutionary pendulum of the hospital experience will, by necessity and demand, return to a more humane base but it may take years.

Being a patient in a hospital is very frustrating and, most of the time, very boring. In the bigger facilities it is very easy to become that number on a wrist band instead of an individual person with needs. I can tell you from years of experience that the patients who maintained a positive attitude are the ones who, not only heal the fastest but also receive the most positive interaction with staff. Making sure that you are recognized as an individual can be as simple as a smile and eye contact. And it is just common courtesy to say please and thank you. Yet another place that your advocate can come in handy if you just don't feel like smiling.

The same holds true for staff. The cheerful bedside nurse of yesterday no longer has the time to give her patients back rubs with the bed bath or sit and visit with the family.   Doctors and nurses have to focus on documentation and look at the computer screens more than they do the patient. But as with the patient, the staff that can maintain a positive attitude, recognizing the humanity curled up in that bed linen and not just the admit number on the wrist band, are the ones that are remembered fondly by the ones they care for.

In any large organization there will be problems. Communication is the biggest culprit here. In American culture it is considered rude to be the "squeaky wheel' but it is your body, your life, that is at stake here. I always told my patients to "squeak away" until they received the attention and the answers they were seeking. I advise you to do the same. In the rushed pace of a modern hospital that may be the only way your get the attention you deserve. Anything that involves your physical well-being makes it your duty as the patient to ask questions and seek answers.

The same holds true for your physicians. Doctors are smart but they don't know everything. The really smart ones are the ones that admit when they don't know it all and will refer you to specialists who may have the answers you need. I cannot emphasize enough the importance of doing your own research into the problems that you are facing, finding all of the possible paths that you want your cure to take, sharing them with friends and family, and being able to discuss your health issues honestly with your physician.   No one has a more personal interest in the recovery of your body than you do. If your Doctor is not receptive to your research into your diagnosis and supplemental treatments that you want to discuss, then it is time to find another Doctor. Find one that respects your right to understand what is happening to your body and will be willing to intercede on your behalf during your hospital stay.

To staff that says, 'The patient isn't always right' I say that you are wrong: The patient isn't always educated fully. Our country prides itself on our laws of self-determination so the decisions that are made by your patient are the ones that are right for them. If you feel they are in error, provide the necessary education to adjust the decisions being made. But bear in mind that the body you are talking about belongs to the patient, not you. They are the ones who will live or die with that body.

If you, as the patient, have problems other than medical ones while you are in the hospital that you wish to have addressed, please be tolerant of the hospital staff. It is not the job of your nurse to fix the TV although she will have someone call maintenance. Issues of entertainment and extra comfort are not foremost in the minds of the hospital staff although they will address them for you when time allows. Quality control issues, such as the melted Jell-O, can probably wait until you are home to be addressed. Take care of your health first and then you can address the problems you saw while you were in the hospital. The Hospital really does want to know your honest opinion of your stay.

They are a competitive business that makes changes every day based on complaints and recommendations from you, their customer.

Try to be patient with the hospital staff. They are notoriously over-worked. Almost everyone that gets into the medical field does so because they care about people and want to help in some way. Sometimes it is a special Thank You from a patient that reminds a very frustrated, tired nurse why she got into this business in the first place and gives her the strength to come back another day. Do not underestimate the power that you, the patient, has when it comes to the moral of the hospital staff. Do not underestimate the power that you have in your own care and the healing process you are undertaking.

I hope this book, even the boring parts, helped make the mystery of how hospitals work easier to understand. Years of working in hospitals and health care did not prepare me for the frustration of being a patient and family member of a patient that I have experienced in the last few years. This book was written in the hope that the information contained in it will help make your stay in the hospital a little less mysterious and a lot less frightening. It is, in no way, meant to serve as medical advice. I wrote this book to, based on my own profession and experiences as a patient and the wife of a patient, offer suggestions on how to make your hospital stay less intimidating. Always, remember to ask questions. Take an advocate with you. And above all else, remember that the primary reason for a hospitals existence is to provide you with a place to stay while large numbers of caring people try to make you feel good again.

www.ingramcontent.com/pod-product-compliance
Lightning Source LLC
Chambersburg PA
CBHW051913170526
45168CB00001B/365